BLOODY
MINDED

BLOODY MINDED

MY LIFE IN CYCLING

ALEX DOWSETT
WITH TOM CONNOLLY

BLOOMSBURY SPORT
LONDON · OXFORD · NEW YORK · NEW DELHI · SYDNEY

BLOOMSBURY SPORT
Bloomsbury Publishing Plc
50 Bedford Square, London, WC1B 3DP, UK
29 Earlsfort Terrace, Dublin 2, Ireland

First published in Great Britain 2023
This paperback edition published 2024

A catalogue record for this book is available from the British Library

Library of Congress Cataloguing-in-Publication data has been applied for

ISBN: PB: 978-1-3994-0641-3; ePub: 978-1-3994-0639-0; ePDF: 978-1-3994-0638-3

2 4 6 8 10 9 7 5 3 1

Typeset in Adobe Garamond Pro by Deanta Global Publishing Services, Chennai, India
Printed and bound in Great Britain by CPI Group (UK) Ltd, Croydon, CR0 4YY

MIX
Paper | Supporting
responsible forestry
FSC® C171272

To find out more about our authors and books visit www.bloomsbury.com
and sign up for our newsletters

*To Ted, and anyone dealt a seemingly bad hand at birth.
It isn't fair, but there's a chance it's an opportunity. So go out there and show
the world what you can do and you may find that that bad hand was the
Royal Flush you never dreamed of.*

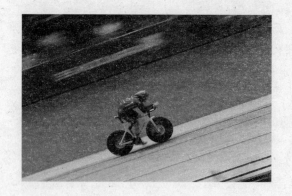

CONTENTS

1

NOT HORRIFIC, JUST TERRIBLE

The Hour Record, 2015

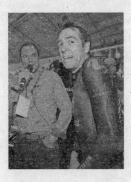

So, this was the sound of 3,000 people losing faith in you. This was the sound of a packed arena beginning to smell failure. There was no anger or disappointment, but something far worse – the sound of silence. And the only thing on earth which naturally fills that silence is self-doubt.

I had put myself in the loneliest place an athlete can be.

It was 2 May, 2015. I was 25 minutes into my attempt to break the World Hour record and the crowd had just realised I was off the pace. The energy had been drained out of them by the possibility that they were watching the most solitary, exposing failure in professional sport.

And they had fallen quiet.

The penalty taker who misses, the marathon runner caught at the last – those things don't come close. If you take on the Hour and fail, there is no one else to blame or praise, no one who has beaten you, no one who has blocked your path to glory. You have failed alone and you have failed entirely, and must face that fact at the lowest physical ebb of your life, one full of pain.

It is one of the phenomena of sport, one of its greatest characteristics, the way that athletes feed off a crowd and the crowd off an athlete. A football team can be trailing and outclassed and one crunching tackle from a journeyman defender ignites the crowd and transforms the game. A tennis player can be on the brink of defeat and playing without rhythm or belief when one glorious, instinctive winning shot makes them suddenly unplayable.

The night before, I had dreamed I was in the middle of my hour attempt and every single seat in the Manchester velodrome was filled with crash-test dummies. They were dressed and sitting forward expectantly, but their faces were blank. I had not produced the power to keep them animated. I walked my bike out of a silent arena. No one could look at me.

Twenty-six minutes in, and my real attempt on the record was a dream come true. The object of the record is to cycle further in 60 minutes than any person has ever done. The apparent simplicity of a ride that takes the body and mind to their deepest reserves and darkest corners makes the Hour one of the most prestigious world records in sport, and utterly unique. Many have failed in attempting it and, if I was in the process of joining them, I was going to be in fine company. But I wanted to put my name among the legends who had broken the Hour – Petit-Breton, Coppi, Anquetil, Baldini, Ritter, Merckx, Moser, Obree, Boardman, Induráin – and become a part of cycling history.

To do it, it's not just that your preparation has to be perfect and every possible legal technical gain found in your bike set-up, skin suit design and your position on the bike (not simply the most aerodynamic but the most aerodynamic position that you can maintain for an hour of increasing physical agony). But on the day your body also has to perform faultlessly while your mind and emotions shut the hell up. You must have a flawless lap-by-lap game plan, then use all your experience and pacing instincts to execute it perfectly.

My mission was simple: ride 212 laps of the 250-metre Manchester velodrome in 60 minutes to go further than the existing record of 52.491 km held by Rohan Dennis.

It is a mission a cyclist undertakes surrounded by friends and supporters, but totally alone. I had a truly exceptional team around me, but was still more exposed than at any other moment in my career; that is the nature of the event. With the Hour, you succeed or you fail; there is nothing else. If you fall short, you find yourself alone, undone, on a small, suddenly claustrophobic, banking track in front of thousands of people who can barely look at you.

And in silence.

I never dreamed of being a pro-cyclist as a kid. I dreamed of a life without the hospital visits and to find something I could be good at. When I did get into cycling and time trialling, the rivalry between Graeme Obree and Chris Boardman was legendary and Boardman had claimed the Hour for a third time. It always seemed to me the ultimate time trial, the holy grail for a TT specialist, but as Obree and Boardman's attempts got more extreme, bikes looked less like bikes and the UCI didn't like it. In 2000 they outlawed the *anything goes* aerodynamic machines and ruled that you had to do the Hour on the same sort of equipment Eddy Merckx rode for his record of 49.431km in 1972. The event went into hibernation because no rider or bike manufacturer wanted to step back in time technically.

Eddy Merckx was the greatest but raced in an era when things were different. He tested positive for doping on several occasions, and was disqualified from races but never banned. I'm playing by a different set of rules, as are the vast majority of riders. In 2014, the UCI announced new criteria for the Hour which allowed modern bikes to be used – aero bars, disc wheels and aero helmets were all permitted – and suddenly my generation of pro cyclists wanted to attack the ultimate TT.

A year earlier, I had signed with the world tour team Movistar. There was history between them and the event with Miguel Induráin's 1994 record. I was adamant that I wanted a shot at the Hour and when Jens Voigt broke the record on 18 September, 2014, covering 51.115km, I started jumping up and down about wanting to do it. It seemed like the natural next step for me. I had won a

TT stage at the Giro in my first year with the team. I had won Gold at the Commonwealth Games and been the national TT Champion. I was fearless, cocky and basically expecting to become an all-time superstar some time soon. And Induráin's legacy meant Movistar had a special place for the Hour in their heart. They responded to me more positively than I was expecting. Eusebio Unzué, the team manager, is a cycling romantic as well as one of the finest minds in the sport, and he saw the opportunity in me for seizing the record.

They booked an hour's training at the London Velodrome and what I thought was a first foray into the possibility of an attempt quickly revealed itself as the start of my team's total commitment to it. As I began to ride around the track, I saw people of note entering the venue to watch me; four from Movistar had made the trip from Spain, the CEO of Endura had come down from Scotland, three people from Canyon in Germany, including Erik Zabel, and a couple from power2max. They had all come to see me do my first training session for a World Hour record attempt that I now realised was no longer just an idea but a reality, and it took me approximately 30 seconds to adjust.

I liked the attention. I realised that Movistar had listened to me banging on about doing the Hour, and had looked at it and decided that in me they had a rider who could. I liked the pressure that came from being selected. That's what I love – being picked.

When you stand in line in the school playground as captains pick teams, being picked last because you're too small or a bit crap provides an obvious motivation. You want to prove people wrong, become sought after. But I was lower in the food chain than that. I wasn't even in the line as a kid. I was watching from the side or sent to the library. Selection means so much to me; by my team, by my country. Movistar didn't back cyclists to do the Hour regularly. They hadn't attempted it for 21 years, and they put their resources and name behind an assault on the Hour only when they believe you can and will become the fastest man on a bike over an hour in history. For all the pressure, and I certainly felt it, I loved being singled out like this, having been singled out in the worst possible way as a kid.

UCI president Brian Cookson declared how happy he was that Dame Sarah Storey and I would be attempting the men's and women's records on consecutive days. Canyon built the bike phenomenally quickly. In December 2014, we did a launch at Rileys Sports Bar in Central London. My bike was unveiled there and it looked awesome. The Speedmax was already the fastest time trial bike out there and Canyon had custom-made me a version of it for the unique demands of the Hour, based on all the wind tunnel work we had done at Mercedes F1. Campagnolo had created a new Pista wheelset with Cult ceramic bearings. By this time, I was obsessing about my attempt and every possible marginal gain, and the first time I saw the bike it filled me with confidence.

If you've saved up and forked out a small fortune on a bike, you know what it's like to admire and covet and want that bike and to consider it an object of beauty that is going to bring pleasure to your life. I was no different. I loved this bike. I loved looking at it. I couldn't wait to get going on it.

I got stuck into training. Movistar booked the Velodrome at Lee Valley for 8 a.m. sessions, which meant 5 a.m. starts for me. The drag of an early alarm clock was nothing new to me, nor was the hushed start to the day, dressing and making coffee in a fug of sleep, and tiptoeing out of the flat without waking my girlfriend. I had been starting my days at this sort of time for much of my life and the feeling was horrible (sometimes feeling weak and nauseous from being woken mid-REM), but I could switch off mentally and make myself do it on autopilot. What helped, on those early drives through the darkness down to East London, was the fact that my old friend Steve Collins was one of my two coaches, and as much as I hated the early starts, I always looked forward to working with him.

I hit all my target numbers in those track sessions, completed every session. But any sense of overconfidence or celebration at doing so was negated by the knowledge that, to break the Hour, hitting your numbers and performing on the bike was just the beginning of the bare minimum requirement. And every minute I spent on the track taught me more about what a lonely event this was going to be, how stripped down and exposing it was compared to a stage race or time trial. Even the outstanding track sessions we responded to with an understated satisfaction. We never interpreted anything as meaning we were knocking it out of the park. We knew the Hour was an event that undid even the best prepared and finest riders. At our most excitable, we responded to a great session by thinking it meant I had half a chance of not fucking it up.

That said, I was in outstanding physical shape and bang on course when I headed out for a training ride with Mark Cavendish on 13 January, 2015, 45 days before the attempt. At 11.50 that morning, Cav tweeted a photo of the two of us out training. By lunchtime, I had a fractured collarbone and was on my way to hospital.

Cav and I had completed a pretty normal ride around the Essex lanes. We had been tearing into it, producing some serious power and egging each other on, but there had been nothing unusual. I was finishing the session with some standing start efforts. They simulate putting your legs under extreme heavy loads, in a big gear, going from inert to pedalling as hard as you can. It was my first start and I put a huge amount of load through the bike – and the group sets aren't built for that. I was in the second pedal stroke when the chain came off. My right foot went from having 1,200 watts on it to having none, very quickly. That threw me forwards and to the right, and I went straight down.

I lay on the road for a few seconds and instinctively reached for my collarbone. I could feel a piece of bone poking up. I knew I was in trouble and when I sat up I was in agony.

The incident was as innocuous as the effects were disastrous. My Hour record was over. It had been scheduled as a live Eurosport event and the broadcast was cancelled. The London Velodrome was let go. The only thing that took my mind off the huge headache I had created for Movistar and for my manager, Sky Andrew, was my fear of the attempt not being rescheduled. Catastrophising is something I do and I devoted the late winter of 2015 to it. I live in a permanent state of expecting to have my sporting life taken away from me because I had to win it for myself in the first place, against all odds.

Good news came soon, though, from Movistar. I was at home doing some planks, testing my collarbone: if you can hold a plank pose then you can use the tribars on a bike and apply pressure through them. In general, I was finding a return to what training I could manage difficult. The Hour seemed to have gone away and suddenly, despite the World Tour, I felt that I had nothing to focus on and fight for. I had been so fit, so ready, and now I was in a no man's land.

Until Movistar called.

'We've all learned so much and come so far, Alex, we can't waste that. You're doing the Hour as soon as you're fit again.'

That was all I needed. My motivation returned in an instant. I threw myself into training. And soon there was another call, from Steve Collins.

'I've got good news and bad news,' he said.

'The bad first, please.'

'London is not available.'

'The good?'

'Manchester is quicker.'

'There's no bad news there,' I said.

Manchester's Velodrome was a second home to me after the thousands of hours I had spent on it during my time at the GB Academy. I was very happy to be returning. They were far more accommodating than London, and it was the track where Chris Boardman had broken the record, which also meant a lot to me.

The new date was set for May and in early spring we headed north. We discovered that Manchester was 10 watts quicker. *This is great, I thought. This is perfect. We're meant to be here.* Weirdly, the track was flatter in Manchester. When you transition from the banking to the straight in London, you seem to lift up a little bit and it shaved a fraction off your speed. You'd have to lean into that and then, as you dropped into the banking, you'd accelerate a bit and correct again. The Hour is not a steady state power profile. You're doing more wattage on the straights than you are on the bankings. The smaller disparity between the power needed on the two in Manchester brought the average power requirement down.

Manchester was where I began to realise that the Hour is not the ultimate time trial after all. It's a different beast. In a TT there are moments of rest, at roundabouts, downhills, in a tailwind. Those don't exist on the track. And in a TT you go as fast as you possibly can. To crack the Hour and not let it crack you, you go as fast as you need.

All the hard work we put into the wind tunnel sessions was not designed to make me faster but to make 52.5km easier. The goal was to bring the power required down. And the power required for the rescheduled attempt kept coming down. If I had started requiring 400 watts, the Manchester track had brought that down to 390. A faster skin suit would get it to 380, faster wheels to 370. That was our rationale: don't make me faster; make the record more achievable.

We tested 14 different skin suits in one day, 53 in total. I was in the tunnel from 8 a.m. to 8 p.m. Endura's suit was sensational and their refusal to settle for anything but the best was one of the most satisfying professional encounters of my career. They would decide that a change to the stitching would make an infinitesimal gain and they'd do it, knowing that every single detail could add up to a world record.

Conti came through with some faster tyres, Campagnolo with faster wheels; both improvements marginal. We freed up all the bearings, optimised with a wax chain, used aero socks which were in their infancy then because you weren't allowed to use overshoes. We had a gold-plated rear sprocket to reduce friction. The bike was silent as I rode it and silence from the bike is as good as it is bad from a crowd. We calculated that a temperature of 30 degrees in the velodrome would bring the watts down further. On my final training session Dad said: 'It's lovely and warm in here' and I laughed. 'Yes, that's not for your benefit, that's for me.'

We had to make the Hour easier, not faster. Movistar were adamant about this in every meeting; 'You break the record and that's it. We're not here to go as fast as we can.' To every degree you go too fast early in the Hour, you suffer and lose distance later. Movistar had put a bucketload of money into the event, organised everything, then reorganised everything. All the sponsors had put money in. They wanted cautious glory, achieved in a grown-up way. Of all those adjectives, *glory* was the only one that got me excited, but I took the counsel of my team and my own coaches. We try to break Rohan's record. We don't try to knock it into orbit.

Movistar wanted the record and were trying to protect me from myself: if you screw up the Hour – not because you fail to break it, but because you mess it up by tearing off too fast and falling short – your reputation and position are hugely damaged. People doubt your ability to think straight and be strategic, which is a huge part of your sport.

You stick to the plan and whatever you do, you don't do a Bobridge.

Prior to my attempt some, like Thomas Dekker, had failed valiantly and by a whisper. Gustav Erik Larsson had failed spectacularly. But no one had done what Jack Bobridge did.

The Hour is an unknown for everyone taking it on. The final 15–20 minutes are, in particular, viewed as uncharted territory for any rider and those like Rohan, Jens and Matthias Brändle were respectful of it and played their attempts down, because there are horror stories. You can't understand in advance quite how it's going to feel or affect you, and why it's not as straightforward as perhaps it ought to be. Eddy Merckx claimed that the Hour had taken a year or two off his life.

Endura had close links to Graeme Obree and said to Movistar, 'Here's Graeme's number, Alex should call him.' But I didn't want to hear how hard it is. It's like giving a pregnant woman the numbers of five women who have been through labour. I tried to avoid talking to anyone who had attempted it. Having spent huge portions of my childhood in pain, I have no fascination with pain as a subject for discussion.

But I had watched all the recent attempts. Dekker missed it by next to nothing, and he'd done so well given he was not a time trialist. Rohan had been brilliantly clinical, so had Brändle. Larsson, I suspect, approached it like a time trial and went in woefully unprepared to ride the track. He's a very smooth time trialist, but it looked like he'd not given it the respect it deserves because he was all over the place. I learned lessons from all of them, but my focus was solely on our strategy, not on anecdotes and horror stories.

That said, there was no avoiding the biggest horror story of all. Jack Bobridge approached the Hour differently. He got a tattoo of a clock on his chest and boasted, 'I'm aiming to set a benchmark that leaves everyone questioning themselves about whether they want to do it or not.'

Well, he did exactly that, but probably not in the way he intended.

In the build-up to Bobridge's attempt and at the same time as I was having a plate drilled into my broken collarbone, Rohan Dennis announced he was going for the Hour – and it was generally accepted that Wiggins would do so too. In Jack's mind, he was going to post an untouchable distance that would make the future attempts by both those greats redundant. He went out of the blocks looking to annihilate the future field, but he came undone and it made for uncomfortable viewing.

To be fair to him, Bobridge went further than Voigt, set a new Australian record and was half a kilometre short of Brändle's record, but he set out a pace to do 55km and failed spectacularly. The only way they could get him off the bike afterwards was by removing the front wheel and have three men hoist him off on to a chair.

'I was in that much pain I couldn't walk. I think it was the closest I could feel to death without actually dying,' he said. It didn't look like an exaggeration.

It was a wake-up call to me and to Movistar, a reminder that you have to respect the Hour as seriously as you respect the mountains or the sea. If you don't, it will chew you up and spit you out. It is a world record that offers the possibility of entering a place of pain that not even an experienced bike rider knows about.

But although Bobridge failed, and latterly – sadly – went off the rails, ending up in prison for drug dealing, he had two qualities that every truly great, pro cyclist needs: ridiculous levels of self-confidence and an ability to embrace pain. I was told that before the 2009 World U23 TT Championships, the three-time world champion Mick Rogers had advised Jack to attack the climb in a lower (easier to pedal) gear on the small chainring, saying, 'You need to do that climb in the little ring,' and Jack replied, 'Not if you're here to fucking win the race.' Mick repeated, 'If you do it in the big ring, you will grind to a halt and pay for it.' Jack dismissed him: 'No, I'm here to win the race.' He did it in the big ring and he won the race, but in every picture of him doing it his eyes were pointing in different directions from the agony. Jack could put himself somewhere that few other riders can.

While it's an unavoidable truth that he became a byword for how not to do the Hour, perhaps I could do with a bit of what Bobridge has from time to time. But you don't want to become a verb in cycling and that's what Bobridge became in our camp. 'We can't do a Bobridge.' Everyone was muttering it. Even Eusebio, my boss, who does not speak a word of English, would walk around saying, 'No Bobridge.'

A lot of science and equipment and expertise precedes an attempt at the Hour in the modern era. But cycling has a habit of bringing you back down to earth. My final warm-up before leaving for the Velodrome took place in the hotel car park. There was nowhere better to do it.

So, under a grey sky, on the tarmac of a car park, beneath the elevated rail line and surrounding tower blocks, sandwiched between our old blue van and a white transit with the words *crusty headfuck* written into the dirt on the rear doors, an elite professional athlete started the process of loosening up his finely tuned body and clearing his mind. And given that most elite cyclists do not have physiques like Zac Efron or Tom Daley (we'd be useless if we did), I must have looked like some skinny eccentric, pedalling and going nowhere in the least exotic of settings, and not like an athlete on the brink – potentially – of making history.

And at the same moment, without me knowing it, the tribars on my bike were being incorrectly adjusted and a skin suit was being unpacked for me that would prove so difficult to get on that two grown men would be needed to zip me into it, leaving my dignity – or what was left of it after a few years on the World Tour – on the floor of the changing rooms.

The life of a professional World Tour cyclist embraces thrill and banality, the glamorous and the drab, the collective and the solitary, and places your chances in the shaky hands of teams that are both state-of-the-art and shambolic. It brings you the adulation of dedicated, fanatical, warm-hearted fans at the same time as a disregard from your employers that can sometimes range anywhere from the dismissive to the abusive. It pinballs you from moments of perfectly organised team logistics that usher you seamlessly through your working life, to periods of total mayhem where you have no idea which country you'll be in next week and if you'll have a job next year. I have been made to feel indispensable and like a piece of dirt by the same bosses in the same week. I have been coached by the best minds in professional sport and left to sort out my own training and diet at my own expense. I've watched grown men crawl out of bed with broken bones, burned skin and internal bruising, and climb back on to the bike for a punishing 200km bike race because they are terrified of not having their contract renewed. The world of professional bike racing is a total shitshow, and I am grateful and privileged to have been a part of it for so many years.

So there was nothing surprising about the fact that, as thousands of people took their seats in the arena above us and the global cycling community trained their eyes on the live coverage of an elite athlete's attempt at a world record, I was naked in the subterranean changing rooms and trying to climb into a skimpy piece of chamois-padded Lycra, ultimately being manhandled and stuffed into it by Simon Smart, one of the finest minds in aerodynamics, and Jim McFarlane, the CEO of Endura.

The skin suit was down to me. Endura had tested 53 versions of it in the wind tunnel with me before we decided that number 52 was the one, but with one final alteration. 'Make the zip as short as humanly possible,' I had told them. Which is why, for a moment in time, these two highly accomplished men had one job, to engage in what would have seemed to a passer-by like a disturbing game of partially naked Twister, forcing my limbs into the right openings and giving me the mother of all wedgies.

Once on, the suit felt superb. It fitted perfectly (well, it would, after 53 versions), offered me serious aerodynamic gains and looked brilliant in the deep dark blue and luminous green of Movistar.

But I was agitated now, the half hour on the turbo-trainer designed to work up a sweat superseded by the battle of Lycra. I was not in the calm, focused state that an assault on the Hour demands. As members of my inner circle came and went, some hand-picked by me, some by my team, the opening of the dressing room door gave snatched hints at the growing noise above me. But when the doors were shut, there was near silence and I could focus on getting my head into the right place, where no self-doubt exists. That has been a difficult place for me to access at times in my career. What I have achieved has been despite an often tormenting brew of strong self-belief in my ability and a deep-rooted expectation that things will go wrong because, at the very top level of cycling, a lot does go wrong, with our bikes and bodies, and with just about every other imaginable factor that can affect your performance. And that is what makes the Hour so seductive. Many of the elements that capsize your cycling dreams are stripped away – other cyclists, to name the principal one – and this makes the task both simple and daunting.

Moments before executing the strategy we had worked on for months, the simplicity of the ride eluded me and I could see only the fear.

Lois, my sister, came to the rescue. She sat quietly opposite me in the changing room, and just her presence allowed me to gather my thoughts and refocus. Soon it was just the two of us, and the whole world seemed to have fallen silent for a few precious seconds until the voice on the stadium tannoy rang out, muted unintelligibly to us but whipping up the crowd, whose voices and stamping feet carried down to us and told me it was time. For a split second I thought I was going to throw up, but then I felt a surge of adrenaline and, instead of nerves, I felt excitement. I was ready. I was not going before a firing squad, I was going before thousands of people who wanted me to succeed. Most of them knew my story, that I might so easily have died in childhood before I ever got to climb on a bike. They knew the improbability of me being here today doing this. They were here because they believed I could become the fastest man on earth on a bike over an hour. They were all on my side.

I reminded myself I was honoured to be here, lucky to be alive. Any cyclist who cannot relish a moment like this does not deserve the chance. Most cyclists who aim for a professional career don't make it. Of those who do, the majority of them have to abandon hope of winning races at the start of their career and become domestiques, worker bees who exist to serve other riders. Most professional cyclists ride more than 10,000km every year in 80–100 race days, spending more than 200 nights in faceless, often shabby hotel rooms shared with a teammate, without winning a single race. One or two cyclists each year will get to attempt the Hour and most of them will fail. I was moments away from my shot at glory; how many people get one of those?

Then I heard exactly what I needed: the sound of my sister's voice, as unflappable and matter-of-fact as if we were going to the supermarket.

'Come on then,' she said.

She stood up, with the permanent expression of slight concern that she has inherited from our mum. I smiled at her and nodded. I stood up too. I took a deep breath and she gave me a hug, then slapped my back as if to tell me to stop dicking about and get on with it. She pushed me out of the changing room and I headed into the underground passageway in which the noise from above grew steadily as I got closer to the entrance to the arena. I was 27 years old and walking to my destiny. At the final doors before the slope up to the inside of the track, I saw on the ceiling in big block letters, the words, *This moment is yours*.

Canyon had made three bikes for me: the training bike, the spare and the race bike. The choreography of the event was that I had to ride the spare bike up a ramp and around half a lap of the track to get to the race bike. As I cycled up the ramp and emerged into the centre of the track, the sound of the crowd in the Velodrome lifted like a single atmospheric swell as people rose to their feet. I took a slow, deep breath into my stomach and chest, and let it out slowly, to keep my composure. I had never experienced an atmosphere like it, because unlike every other bike race I had been in, these people were here to watch me, and only me. It was more like being a rock star than a professional cyclist, except that a rock star can go with the flow, change tactics, make and get away with small mistakes, start late and finish late. My performance had to be disciplined and perfect in every detail, which is probably why you don't hear Hour record cyclists enter a velodrome screaming, 'GOOD EVENING MANCHESTER!'

I cruised the track on the spare bike. In the VIP section inside the track, I spotted a few familiar faces, but deliberately didn't settle on any or make eye contact. Most of my friends were there, but I knew I couldn't afford to break my focus by engaging with them. I caught sight of my teammate, Adriano Malori, the other time trial specialist at Movistar. He was a better time trialist than me and from the fact that he had come to support me I drew strength – another marginal gain when every one of them, both mental and physical, helps. On the other side of the track I saw a wall of people looking down on me, people just like my parents and my friends, working people with a love of cycling. I didn't know them but they all felt familiar, the sort of people I like chatting to and doing selfies with at races, the cycling fans who have always treated me well and to whom I owe a lot.

I had raced in front of packed stadiums, but as the pressure of being the sole focus hit me so did an almost comic realisation of just how bad failure here would taste. It's a kind of privilege to be at the centre of something that matters enough to scare the shit out of you.

I came to a halt and dismounted the spare bike, which was put on show along with the training bike in the track centre. Tomas, the Movistar mechanic, helped me on to the race bike. He was a lovely, calming, ever-enthusiastic presence and exactly the person I wanted there with me in the final, tense seconds of build-up. He squeezed the back of my neck and wished my luck. Now I was alone on the bike and I immediately saw that the handlebars had been set up wrong.

My immediate reaction was an unreasonably calm one. *Well, that's not what I've been training on for the last five months but it's going to look seriously unprofessional if everyone watching sees me ask for an Allen key and I start messing with the bike.*

But then I felt a panic rising in me.

Shit.

For a few seconds, probably half a minute in total, the sound of everyone around me fell away and I was in my own world, where my thoughts and my breathing were giants in my head, obscuring everything else. *How to deal with these bars? How the fuck could this be happening?*

In fact, it was easy enough to guess. I have my tribars tipped slightly towards each other because it helps me bring my shoulders in and my hands close. I think what had happened was the UCI had checked the dimensions of the bike and probably found it a little too long. It would have only been by a maximum of a centimetre. It would've been something the team did not need to worry me with, but when they'd moved the bars back, they had straightened them.

I didn't really want to get into changing the set-up, given that what I'm like with alterations means these things can take a while. But, at the same time, everything was meant to be perfect. I decided I just wanted to get the fuck on with it and for once I overrode that tinker man part of me and thought, *I'll deal with it.* I felt that the delay, the loss of momentum that fixing the bars would cause, would be a greater loss than the incorrect position of the bars. Welcome to the inside of a world tour cyclist's head, where everything in your life is the weighing up of a marginal loss or gain, of a watt of power or a hundredth of a second. The bars being wrong versus the stress of altering them in the middle of the arena. The weight gain of an extra slice of toast versus the mental wellbeing of enjoying your breakfast. It never stops.

I shrugged it off, which is not like me. And it helped, it got me into a good mental state. *Fuck it. It doesn't matter if I don't let it matter. Let's just get on the bike and do the thing.*

The arena fell silent the moment I got on to the race bike. The MC, Joe Fisher, announced we were 45 seconds from the start. The silence was total and unnerving. They couldn't have been more quiet if I had died (which might have got the odd cheer; I wasn't everyone's cup of tea at Movistar) and I knew I had to deal with it before any nagging doubt filled the void. I tried to focus on a perfect start. We had learned our strategy for the first lap from Matthias Brändle. The start of the Hour is extreme due to a static start in the big single gear that you use for the whole race. You don't want to give away time by getting up to speed too slowly, but you can't burn excess strength by sprinting. The first few seconds are such a small part of the race, but hugely significant and potentially damaging.

In training, my starts were always too slow – at around 26, 27, 28 seconds. I was standing on the pedals for half a lap. I had studied Brändle, who was in the saddle and on the aero bars within a quarter of a lap and dismissed it. 'He's got no idea,' were the words I used to Steve Collins. But I wasn't hitting my times in training, so we tried Brändle's method and I immediately hit a 24-second first lap using far less power. Matthias knew what he was doing and I took a valuable lesson from him.

I was now less than 10 seconds away from putting it into action. The timer counted down the final 5 seconds. I rose up off my saddle and, a split second before the clock started, I pushed my body forward and the crowd erupted, slapping their clappers together, roaring, cheering. For a moment, their noise and the effort of pushing through the lead-heavy gear created a sensation of inertia.

I'm not moving!

It was a fraction of a second, no more, just another slither of opportunity for doubt and panic to try and find a way into me, but in reality my start had been perfect. I was in the saddle almost instantly and the movement of the bike was smooth into the first bend. I was half a second too fast on the first lap. The crowd knew it and went even more nuts. *They can't keep this up*, I thought, *and neither can I*. In the build-up I had talked about the Hour being an unknown quantity, but it was only now, in those rowdy first few laps, that I understood the extent to which any man or woman attempting this record enters uncharted territory. In training, you'll never do the full hour. You do not truly know what effect the full 60 minutes will have on your body and mind.

I reminded myself how simple the team plan was. Do a 25-second first lap, and then do 17-second laps after that, and you'll break the Hour record. Steve was trackside feeding me my lap times. If I had just done a 17-second lap, he'd put his hand out flat. If I came past having done 16.8, he'd point two fingers upwards; and if I'd done a 17.1, he'd put one finger down. My target was to see either his flat hand, or one or two fingers pointing in the sky. I did not want to see any pointing down at any moment in the race. As a team, we had adopted a zero-ego approach. No strutting, no over-exuberance, no showing off or pushing it. We had a conservative schedule in place to beat Rohan Dennis' record. It didn't matter if we did it by a metre or a kilometre.

I got into a good rhythm and the first half of the race went quickly for me. At nine minutes, I hit 52 km/h and the crowd erupted. I hadn't expected the physical discomfort to kick in so early, but when it did I realised that the pain was like grief: you ride with it, you live with it, you don't try to banish it because if you could do an Hour without profound physical pain, then you wouldn't be human. If you love someone and don't feel loss when they go, then you're not human either. The Hour is an experience of pure physical pain. That fact is the one thing that unites all of us who have attempted it, from every era. There's simply no choice. If I want to be the fastest man ever over 60 minutes, it's going to hurt.

What was good was that, despite the pain, I was in a balanced state where I was aware of the crowd, the MC and, occasionally, friends and family inside the track, but none of these things penetrated my thinking or cadence. For 25 minutes I was metronomic. It's not effortless or without suffering, but it's a perfectly balanced state, where your training, your mental strength, your fitness and your desire are an exact match for the pain and the fear of failure. Neither side wins out. You are riding in a neutral state.

And that's what I did for almost the first half of the race until that moment at 25 minutes when I became aware of something having changed around me, and I looked up and glimpsed the blank faces. And as I swept around the arena, it was as if I was waving a wand that magicked a deafening silence on the place.

I was behind and the crowd had lost faith. What had happened? I had been hitting all my lap times. Hadn't I? Or had I stopped looking at Steve? Had my neutral state to mentally deal with the physical pain simply turned into falling off the pace?

I was lost.

And a voice came into my head out of the distant past.

We'd rather you played chess.

I had not expected that.

It was the voice of the specialist who had looked after me as a kid. When my Dad told him that I wanted to race bikes, he said, 'We'd rather he played chess.'

Maybe he was right, I thought, as I did another lap in stony silence. *Maybe I should be playing chess.*

But the reality was that I had been behind Rohan Dennis from the start and was meant to be. We had a different game plan to Rohan. But the crowd had seen that I was 24 seconds off his record at 25 minutes and lost their nerve, and that threw me.

What was I thinking? I should be playing chess.

It seemed like a lifetime, like time had stopped, but in reality the silence that fell on the Velodrome, and the loss of nerve, lasted only a few minutes. But that is the nature of the Hour. Everything seems different to a race. Every second seems like a lifetime. But the reality is that you perform on the training and years of experience and savvy, and the physical and mental torment does not shake you from your purpose or your game plan. Not if you're any good.

I upped the pace, but did it fractionally, enough to reassure the crowd without altering the game plan. It was my way of regaining full consciousness and control. Rohan Dennis had started quick, got quicker for half an hour and then slowed in the second half. My game plan was different, a flat line on a graph compared to Rohan's midway peak. Now, I was being a rock star, sticking to the plan but playing the crowd by giving them a bit of what they needed.

Which was confidence. Confidence in me. That they were not watching a failure.

At 32 minutes, the MC, Joe Fisher, wound the crowd back up, telling them I was making ground on Rohan Dennis' record. The crowd saw me take another second back from Rohan and responded, sitting forward, shouting, roaring, reanimating. My lap times went through the roof, five or six tenths of a second too fast. Steve Collins got agitated trackside. I was saying all the right things to myself – *stay disciplined, calm down, ignore the crowd* – but the whole new level of noise in the place had thrown me off and for a couple more laps I couldn't bring my speed down. The trouble was, I loved the crowd and I was excited about getting them back off their seats and wanted to keep them there. When my lap splits plummeted to 16.2, instead of holding eight fingers up, Steve just screamed at me, 'SLOW THE FUCK DOWN.'

I brought it back in.

Don't do a Bobridge, Alex. Do what you're here to do.

It was my best period on the bike that day, because it's much harder to rein it in like that and come down to a fractionally slower speed than it is to ask your body to go flat out and produce whatever it can.

I was just over halfway; the crowd were back with me and I was learning fast on the job. But there was a long way to go and, despite the cool, set, unchanging appearance of my face and position, my heart was racing and I felt shaky, realising that a few overexcited laps could capsize months and months of plotting and training.

We'd rather you played chess.

It was like a warning to me. *You're not really meant to be here. There's still time to mess this up. And when that happens, you'll wish you'd never got on a bike.*

The Hour record has many ways of defeating you and one is the apparent simplicity of it. Ride as far as you can in an hour; straightforward, right? But in practice, it is a test that demands you keep perfect physical and mental discipline for 60 minutes while experiencing a gradually intensifying physical pain which reminds you, lap after lap, that however brilliantly you ride, you don't get to finish any sooner.

There is no respite and no welcome distraction. You have the black, painted line on the inside of the track to watch your front wheel sticking to – and nothing else, no bends or climbs or views to help pass the time, no downhills to steal a moment's rest as you freewheel. The Hour is a challenge apart and the ways in which it is not like a time trial are brutal. The repetition of the same 250-metre track leaves room for all sorts of weird things to play on your mind and try to capsize you. The relentlessness of the power effort is an attack on your body strength, which no time trial quite sets you up for.

Thomas Dekker, who described his attempt earlier that year as 'the worst hour of my life', talked about having a real rough patch at 40 minutes. I was waiting for that to bite me, but 40 minutes came and went and I felt steady. I glanced up at the clock at 43 minutes and thought to myself, *I'm okay*. I began to lose my immediate awareness of the physical pain and to feel hyper-aware of everything else. I should have tucked my head down more than I did, but lap by lap, from glances up, I built a map of where everyone was inside the track – my team, my dad, my sister and girlfriend, my mates. And now my brain created a strange sensation of two versions of me on the bike, one in the aero position, powering on, and the other riding sat up with my hands off the bars slapping my thighs as they rose on the pedal, like a cocky street kid. The cocky version of me was drinking in this extraordinary event and allowing the support of the crowd to fill every cell in my body and pore in my skin. He was grinning from ear to ear, an expression almost identical to the grimace of the real me on the bike. The aero version of me was sticking to the pacing strategy and dealing with the pain in my legs, arse and lungs.

Joe Fisher, a big unshaven bear of a man with his microphone, was working the crowd, inciting them with updates on where I was in relation to Dennis' record. And the weird thing is, I was listening to him, the same way I was picking out faces in the crowd. For all but the occasional moment I was head down, powering the bike, totally focused, nailing the game plan, and yet I was also getting this close to an out-of-body experience of the event, the arena, in its mad, crazed, loud entirety.

It was as close to being a spectator of my own performance as I ever got, because the actual riding had taken on the illusion of being comfortable. And, of course, it wasn't comfortable. At 40 minutes, I entered the unknown territory of the Hour in the greatest agony I had ever experienced on a bike. The build-up of lactic acid and the time spent in the fixed riding position was taking its toll. It was a deep, all-encompassing pain, not sharp, not shooting, but draining of all your strength. My shoulders were tired and holding my position on the black line on the banking was now an effort. My mouth was horribly dry. My leg muscles were screaming at me, so I tried to ignore them and focus on my heart and lungs pumping, but the moment I did that they screamed at me too: *Get off the bike, just get off the bike.* My mind moved between different areas of pain until I found myself in that incredible place where your mind obliterates the pain and your body is continuing to produce the goods because the lessons ingrained in you psychologically and physiologically during thousands upon thousands of hours of training and living with pain are now running the show. It is, quite simply, the moment when you are being the greatest version of your athletic self. It is a kind of rapture. If you achieve this, you have a chance of taking the Hour. But no more than a chance.

You cannot do the Hour without feeling pain, but if you do it with all your mental strength about you, if you are lucky enough to feel brave and strong that day, the pain doesn't defeat you. It registers but it doesn't win. And you begin to feel untouchable. That extraordinary sensation swept me into the last 10 minutes as I slashed the gap on Rohan's record down to 2.8 seconds, causing another rise in volume from the crowd. I was beginning to enjoy it and the crowd were finding new levels beyond what I had presumed must be their peak, making noise like nothing I had ever known.

But Steve Collins was worried. It was his job to be. He marched down to the trackside and shouted, 'ALEX! KEEP YOUR HEAD DOWN!'

He knew it was still a 10-minute effort and you can do a lot of damage to yourself in 10 minutes. My laps crept down to 16.8, 16.7, and he was still reining me in, protecting me from myself. He was a fantastic judge, allowing me to dial it up a little bit but keeping me on a leash. On lap 180, 51 minutes into my ride, my time went below the current record. I was ahead of Rohan Dennis for the first time and getting faster. The atmosphere was becoming carnival like, a bit unhinged, with people thumping the hoardings, stamping their feet, using the clappers like drumsticks, roaring and cheering. It made me feel powerful to be able to ignite this response from them, to be able to obliterate the pain. Even with five minutes to go I felt that I was holding back, sticking to the plan. Then, with two minutes left, Steve stepped back from the very edge of the track. No more hand signals.

'Off you go!' he shouted.

He smiled at me for the first time in five months. He's an ugly bastard, but for that moment, with that smile, as he let me loose, he was the most beautiful man in the world.

All hell broke loose at that point. I felt as ecstatic as Joe Fisher and the crowd sounded. Thousands of Canyon-branded clappers shook and waved on the home straight. Bodies strained forward towards the track from the seating. Mouths seemed suspended open, cheering, eyes bright, faces excited, full of belief. They were giving all this to me – and I was creating this in them. *What a feeling!* Smiling faces everywhere. I glimpsed Sky Andrew jumping up and down on the spot in the in-field, like an excited kid. I did the last 5 laps at 15.5, which was monstrously fast. I knew we'd done it. I was so ahead that it would have been very difficult to lose. I felt phenomenal. I felt I had more.

On lap 210, with 45 seconds left, the entire crowd rose to their feet. It was one of the most breathtaking, humbling moments of my life. Steve clenched his fist and screamed my name as I passed him; I drilled down faster and faster, trying to hit 53km/h. The whistle went, the crowd lifted the roof, I punched my fist and rose up on my seat for the first time in an hour and, as I circled the track slower and slower, I tried to take in the reaction of the crowd, which was almost frightening to me. I owed them so much. I removed my helmet, tossed it to Tomas as I passed and punched the air repeatedly as I glided past the crowd, thanking them, waving to people and grimacing with the effort not to burst into tears. I still looked as if I was in pain. I was not. I was, quite simply, overwhelmed.

As I came around to where Steve Collins was standing, I sat back and clasped my hands together – as if in prayer? I don't know what I was doing. I was incapable of expressing myself. But I nearly lost my shit as Steve opened his arms out to me. We made a pretty good fist of embracing each other given that I was moving forwards on a bike and he was standing still. How he didn't bring me down, I don't know. And maybe it's a good thing that I was still moving because had I stopped there in Steve's arms, I simply would not have known how to begin to express my thanks to him.

I went along a line of outstretched hands, slapping them all, trying to smile but too tired and emotional to do so. I did a final slow lap for the crowd, waving to them, trying – and, I fear, failing – to convey my thanks. And then I came to a halt in the embrace of Tomas and climbed off the bike. For a second, Tomas held the bike and we looked at each other. He has a kind face, he's loyal and attentive, entirely without ego and he was so happy for me. I gave him the most barely perceptible of nods, it was all I could muster, and I knew he understood how grateful I was to him.

Suddenly, ridiculously, I felt fresh, such is the physical effect of triumph. Had I failed with the exact same physical effort, I would have collapsed. Unrehearsed, without thinking about it, I took the bike back from Tomas and held it up above my head. The crowd loved this, but not half as much as Canyon loved it.

I handed the bike over to Tomas again, then turned and embraced my sister and my girlfriend. I squeezed them tight. Lois patted my back. It was a tiny gesture that said everything we know about each other, that we've been on a journey together since our childhoods, that we've endured the challenges together and we share the moments of joy. I left the track that had served me so well and stepped into the in-field, into the embrace of Sky Andrew. I said a few private words to him as we hugged, a message of thanks and admiration. Then the grinning, happy face of my boss at Movistar, Eusebio, as he embraced me and slapped my back, exuding the pure love of this sport that man has and which has sustained him across his long career.

A journalist stuck a microphone in my face and asked me about the pain.

'I was expecting horrific and it was just terrible,' I said.

That comment aside, my memories of the immediate aftermath are of emotions, not words or physical tiredness. Winning a race is one thing; finishing a race and knowing you are a world record holder, that you have written your name into your sport's history, is something else. And it takes a while to sink in. In the meantime, pure emotion fills the void created by exhaustion and incomprehension. And it's not as if I can even break down the emotion. Joy? Relief? Gratitude? Well, yes, all of those, but for now they were all rolled into one tidal wave of happiness that was so strong it was impossible to resist.

I'm not one of those people who feels indestructible in victory. With an illness like mine, you never feel indestructible. But I did feel that a lot of luck and hard work had put me in the saddle of a beautiful, record-breaking bike instead of in the wheelchair that was once upon a time predicted for me. And I will always be proud of the fact that on 2 May, 2015, I was in such phenomenally good physical shape that I was able to enjoy the Hour. To the same extent that Jack Bobridge's body was entering hell, I was floating. My prize for all my hard work, for being back in the saddle within days of breaking my collarbone, for insisting that my own people, the ones who had always been there for me, were as central to the attempt as Movistar were, my reward for being loyal and fit was that I got to enjoy every single second of the closing stages.

I looked for Dad. Suddenly, I was desperate to find him. I remember saying, 'I need to get to Dad' to someone and at that moment he came through the mass of bodies in the middle of the track. We embraced and clung on to each other, gripped each other tight. His voice straining from the effort not to cry, he said, 'Alex, Alex. I love you, boy. I love you.'

And yet, the person who most deserved to share that moment with me and Dad wasn't there. The UCI have to approve the date so that it doesn't clash with the Grand Tours and when we rescheduled the attempt in Manchester, the only date we could do clashed with Mum being on a cruise in Norway with some girlfriends. She was adamant that she'd cancel her holiday, but one of the friends going with her had been through a terrible time and needed her. And I also started to believe that her cancelling for me would be a bad omen.

'Mum, if you cancel, I probably won't break the record. You've got to go. That's how you can help me.'

So, Mum, wasn't there. It was incredibly unfair on her because she had always been there with me and for me. She was out on the North Sea, alone in her cabin waiting for the phone to ring, which it did within 10 minutes of me getting off the bike.

'Yes?' she said, her voice trembling and sounding a million miles away, which is how she was feeling. 'Yes?'

This was the voice of the woman who gave birth to me and then went through hell as she watched me become a very sick child. This was the woman who had done everything for me.

'I've done it, Mum.'

And that was the most magical moment of all. She wept and I thanked her for giving me this life, for nursing me and pushing me, and turning me into a world record holder – and the only elite athlete in the world with haemophilia.

2

THE DAY MY DAD STOPPED WHISTLING

Diagnosis, 1990

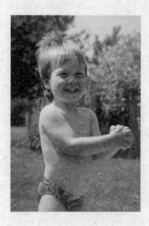

I was born in 1988, with the need for some intervention: forceps, suction and a sodding great bruise on my head. But the bruise faded and no one thought anything of it.

Mum was a hairdresser. Dad had raced cars and was setting up his own business. They both loved their work and each other, and starting a family was a long anticipated and natural next step. Home was the Chelmsford area of the most maligned county in England: Essex.

Mum and Dad had had a lot of fun together and now they had me, a chubby little baby, to dote on. They felt like the luckiest of people. *Chubby* is a word that comes up a lot when anyone who was there describes my start in life. And given that I was a bonny chap and my parents were active people, prone to happiness and having a good time, it would have been hard for them to believe that there could be anything wrong. But as a toddler, when I cruised the family home in Essex in my baby walker, demonstrating an early love of speed that Dad would happily take credit for, Mum found herself taking me repeatedly to the baby clinic to show the health visitor bruises around my midriff and the way in which her picking me up would leave handprints on my skin.

'Oh, he just bruises easily. Don't worry.'

But she did worry, about my bruising and also that someone would think she was hitting me. She kept taking me back and after one of these appointments the health visitor said, 'If you're so worried, take him to the doctor.'

So, Mum moved on to annoying him instead of her.

'He's just a little boy that bruises easily,' the GP said. 'He'll grow out of it.'

When I learned to walk, the falls and bumps that are a natural part of the process left me with huge bruises on my knees, so I would crawl instead. If the bruise was particularly painful, I would move like a crab on my hands and feet, bum stuck in the air, to avoid my knees touching the floor. This was a constant in my life until I was 17 months old and Mum decided she had had enough of being dismissed as a classic, overreacting, first-time parent.

'Do you realise what you'll be putting Alex through with a blood test?' The GP said. 'It's not like a prick on the finger, it has to be done intravenously.'

Mum insisted. She knew there was something wrong and feared it might be leukaemia. The doctor threw the slip of paper across the table at her. 'If you want put him through that, then you do it.'

From Mum's perspective (she remembers and will never forget) and from mine (I don't remember, but Mum has described the scene) the blood test was as bad as the GP had warned. It took half an hour to find a vein they could get into. I went to pieces, screaming, sobbing – and Mum fell apart too seeing how terrified I was of the needle.

As we left the surgery I tripped up and fell over and started bleeding from the lip. Back home, I bled from the lip periodically for the rest of the day. The bleed was coming from the fenulum, the little piece of skin that attaches the top lip to the gum. Mum and Dad put me to bed once the bleeding finally stopped. They checked on me a couple of times. I was asleep and calm. When they turned in for the night, they checked on me again and found me lying in a large pool of blood, big enough to cover most of the pillow. I was fast asleep. It was 10.30 on a Friday night. The emergency doctor came out and stemmed the bleeding. Mum and Dad explained everything that had been happening.

'It's possible,' the doctor said, 'that he's going to be a little bleeder. But I don't think so because it's so rare.'

My dad said, 'What do you mean?'

'The very worst thing it could be is haemophilia.'

That was the first time it was said to them in relation to their child, the word that would define the next years of our lives.

Mum knew what she wanted from an early age. At 13 she went through all the local hairdressers in the *Yellow Pages* until one of them gave her a Saturday job. When she was old enough, they gave her an apprenticeship and she became what she had always wanted to be, a hairdresser, in her hometown of Southend. She fell in love with Dad and they dreamed of having a family. That's the young woman who was listening to this doctor, now being told that her happy-ever-after was no longer a shoo-in.

I was admitted to hospital for more blood tests that were hugely distressing for my parents to witness. The prospect of a diagnosis that would make this sort of experience a regular part of life was unthinkable. I would stare at them as the needles went in with an expression that said, 'Why are you letting this happen?' and it haunted them.

On the Monday night our GP came to find my parents in the hospital, to break the news to them face to face.

'Your son is a haemophiliac. He has the most common form of the condition, haemophilia A. It means he lacks the eighth stage of the blood-clotting process.'

They looked at him and Dad says he was just thinking that, perhaps, *common* might mean *not so bad*, when the doctor added, 'The version of haemophilia Alex has is the most severe. I want to be straight with you. It's about as bad as it gets.'

The fate of any parent whose world is turned upside down by their child's diagnosis is a crash course in a subject they would prefer not to know about. My parents discovered that haemophilia is an inherited disorder, but one which occurs only about 50% of the time. While people assume that hereditary means it is something the family are prepared for, the reality for us was that I was the first in the family. When I had started to bruise and bleed, my parents had no reason to think one of them was carrying the haemophilia gene.

One of them turned out to be Mum. And given the hurt she has suffered believing she 'gave' me haemophilia, I would give anything for that not to be how it works. But an unaffected father and a mother carrying the haemophilia gene have a 50% chance of having a son with haemophilia, and I drew the straw. I am not alone; 1 in 10,000 people have haemophilia, most of them boys.

So why do I say I drew *the straw*, not *the short straw*? There are a few reasons, and they'll become clear, but I'll start with this one: if you're my age and a haemophiliac, you can either rue the bad luck of being the 1 in 10,000 or you can focus on the fact that until the last couple of generations, your life expectancy would have been the teenage years.

When a haemophiliac bleeds, a lack of key proteins means the normal blood-clotting process doesn't kick in, the bleeding doesn't stop and, without medication, the person bleeds to death. That weekend of my diagnosis, I was kept in hospital to control the bleed and, having lost so much blood, I received my first blood transfusion. It was 1990, not the ideal date in history for regular blood transfusions. And it didn't seem to have worked. I was still looking extremely pale when my parents returned to me, but probably not a pale as them. And I was still bleeding. Potentially, to death.

This is what prompted the doctors to give me my first injection of Factor VIII. Dad describes it as being like flicking a switch. The bleeding from my mouth stopped instantly. This was the start of a beautiful friendship between Factor VIII and me. Next stop was the Royal London Hospital in Whitechapel, where I was put under the care of the haematologist, Dr Brian Colvin, with whom my parents experienced the next moment of horror.

'It says here that baby Alex was a forceps and suction delivery,' Dr Colvin said.

'Yes.'

He asked them for a full description of the birth, and the scale and nature of the bruising it caused to my head. The more he heard, the more concerned he became.

'How is Alex's developmental progress?' he asked.

'How do you mean?' Dad said.

'You mean he might be brain damaged,' Mum said.

Given the nature of my delivery, I could easily have had a bleed on the brain from the delivery. There was no way Dr Colvin could disguise his concerns about this or prevent my parents from two days of agonising wait as the Royal London carried out neurological tests. They came back all clear. I was okay. And with 48 hours of frantic reading up on the literature about haemophiliacs and brain bleeds under their belt, Mum and Dad knew how lucky we were on that score.

That scare helped them, though. As they took me home and faced life with a sick child, they already had a sense that this could have been worse.

Dad wanted to know everything from the start, not to be drip-fed. He wanted to plot the future out. Mum wanted to learn as she went along. The two of them were happy to approach it differently. They didn't feel pressure to react to my illness in the same way. And they both agreed 100 per cent on one thing: that coming to terms with my illness was easy in comparison to watching my life turn into a series of attempts to get needles into my young, veinless skin. Maybe it would have helped them back then if they had known that, by introducing me to the experience of regular, intense pain, they were laying the perfect foundations for training to be a pro cyclist.

And, then again, maybe not.

They had a lot going on. Mum's dad had just died and so too had one of Dad's best friends. Then Mum realised that not being able to take a blood sample from her father meant we couldn't trace the genetic link. She fell into a depression. Dad was swamped with work on the new business he had set up following his retirement from motor racing. In those dark days, as Mum struggled to come to terms with what she saw as her having given me an illness, and losing her dad, she noticed how quiet the house was. The laughter between them had gone, replaced by doubt about the future. The boisterous playing, and toddler fun and silliness, with me was on hold as I recovered from my worse bleed and the needle-fest of my diagnosis. And Dad had stopped whistling. Mum had always known where in the house or the garden he was because he was whistling. It sometimes drove her nuts, but suddenly the house felt different without it. The fun and the laughter and the silly games – and the happiness – soon returned, but the whistling didn't. It was something he never did again. It's a silly thing, but to Mum it always marked that time when their lives changed.

My parents loved the haemophilia nurse who was assigned to us. She was called Wanda and she told Mum and Dad about meetings for parents of haemophiliacs. They went along to one and it was not their style. They found it depressing, all doom and gloom. They had a group of parents telling them, as first-timers, how bad things were going to get. One man talked at length about the nightmare of your child's first teeth falling out and the bleeds then. My parents came away from it adamant they would not go again.

They weren't in denial and they weren't being superior. They just didn't want to spend their spare time talking about haemophilia. They would face each challenge as it came up, they would do everything they could for me, but they would not go to another one of those meetings.

Soon after that, they did agree to visit to a family whose son had haemophilia, as it had been arranged by Wanda, who thought it might be helpful for them because these parents were such positive people. Their son was older, so they could share a lot of what the next few years might be like for me. They rang the doorbell and, as they waited, they saw a wheelchair in the porch. My mum broke down.

'Is this what Alex's life will be?' she asked Dad.

The parents were lovely, but it was another demoralising evening that left Mum and Dad with the impression that a wheelchair would be inevitable for me, eventually. But my parents weren't wired to look at life that way. They decided to cut themselves off.

'We'll tread our own path,' Dad said.

'We are not going to live our lives waiting for the next bleed,' Mum said. 'And neither is our son.'

They decided to raise me how they thought best, to make it up as they went along and admit their mistakes along the way. This decision was one of the countless gifts they have given me.

In the early years of my life, synthetic Factor VIII was not available, so you got your Factor VIII from blood transfusions. Those haemophiliacs who were put on to prophylaxis (preventative treatment) rather than being cared for in hospital when a bleed occurred (reactive treatment) were, it turned out, being exposed to the risk of blood infected with HIV or Hepatitis C.

By the time I went under Dr Colvin, he and the rest of the medical community were increasingly aware of the risks of infection. The Hepatitis C virus was finally identified in 1989, when I was one year old. HIV had been identified as infecting blood plasma earlier in the decade. Much of the blood product administered to haemophiliacs in the United Kingdom was imported from abroad, especially from the United States.

In his witness statement to the Infected Blood Enquiry in March 2020, Dr Colvin said: 'It was clear by the end of 1984 that the risk of HIV infection was substantially greater from commercial as opposed to UK sourced plasma concentrate. However, it is now known that, by 1985, HIV had entered the British donor pool and HIV infection did occur. Had self-sufficiency in Factor VIII concentrates production been achieved the number of patients infected with HIV would have been reduced. This was not a wholly avoidable disaster, as has been suggested, even by our own government.'

Despite the pressure to put boys like me with the most severe form of Haemophilia A on to preventative treatment in the form of transfusions of Factor VIII from donated blood plasma, I benefited from Brian Colvin's conservative approach. And when I say that I benefited, I mean that it probably saved my life.

There was another element that possibly saved me and that was timing. Mum and Dad were married for 12 years before they had me. They waited so that Dad could concentrate on his motor racing career. He was with Toyota and rising up the ladder, trying to get into Formula One. Mum's career was established and she loved her job, but she knew Dad's would be short-lived and she wanted to let him go as far as he could as a racing driver before they started a family.

The campaign group *Factor VIII*, a non-profit organisation run by and for those impacted by Hepatitis C- and HIV-infected blood products in the 1970s and 1980s, has a memorial page on its website. What the faces and names on it remind me of is that thousands of people died because they had haemophilia but not from haemophilia. They died from medicine. The blood that was put into them to save their lives killed them. One of the current board members of *Factor VIII*, Lauren Palmer, saw both her parents die when she was nine years old. Her dad, a haemophiliac, was infected with Hep C and HIV from a blood transfusion and he unwittingly infected Lauren's mum; they died within a week of each other.

Had I been born a few years earlier, before my specialist became aware of infection, I might well not be here today. Thousands of haemophiliacs born in the years before me are not. Dr Colvin lived the nightmare of knowing he had unintentionally given some haemophiliacs HIV and Hep C via infected blood products. I arrived in the eye of that storm and came out of my childhood virally clear: I dodged a bullet because he delayed my change to prophylactic treatment.

But this approach also meant that I was prone to bleeds, sometimes serious ones. My sister Lois was born on 3 November, 1991 when I was three. Soon after she arrived, mum came into my room to get me up for nursery and found me standing in the middle of the room as if my foot was glued to the floor.

'Mummy, I can't walk.'

That trip to hospital is one I remember vividly. The doctors could not get a needle into my veins, which is not to say they weren't putting needles into me, they just couldn't draw blood. Three different doctors tried, four times each. Medics were allowed four attempts to try to find a child's vein, after which the risk of their stress causing a mistake was deemed too great, so another medic would step in and try. Twelve times I had a needle put in me and each time I became more upset, my parents became more distressed and even the medical staff got agitated. When a toddler gets distressed, the veins dilate and even a decent-sized vein, which toddlers aren't renowned for, gets smaller and injecting becomes even harder.

All of which explains why a classic behavioural trait in haemophiliac children aged four upwards is to hide their bleeds. Kids don't want the needle, so they fake being okay.

Thus, my life hung in the balance between the risk of death or serious harm through internal bleeding, and the risk of death by infection with HIV or Hepatitis C.

'Because,' my dad jokes, 'having haemophilia isn't enough.'

I was hitting my stride when it came to hiding bleeds by the time we went on a family holiday to Lanzarote, when I was five. One evening, as we left a restaurant, my parents noticed that I was dragging my foot, trying to hide the fact that I couldn't lift it. Mum attempted twice to inject me with Factor VIII, but couldn't get into a vein. My grandma was with us and looked after Lois while Mum and Dad set off with me in search of the hospital. We drove around but couldn't find it. Dad stopped to ask a crowd of people on a street corner for directions.

'Our boy,' he said. 'We need a hospital.'

A woman approached the car. She, like everyone in the group, was grubby from, it would turn out, a day working in the potato fields. She looked in at me, crying with pain on Mum's lap and climbed into the car.

'I show you,' she said.

She was called Victoria and she came into A & E with us and offered to stay and translate. The bleed was getting worse, the pain like a snapped bone. A doctor came in, who spoke as little English as my parents did Spanish. Mum got my Factor VIII out.

'Hemofílico.' She pointed to my veins and to the medicine.

The doctor put the Factor VIII aside and, according to our translator, said she wanted to take a picture of his ankle tomorrow. He would stay the night, in a ward.

Mum said to Victoria, 'No X-rays. Urgent. Urgent.'

Suddenly, Victoria became hysterical, shouting at the doctor in Spanish. The doctor stormed off. After that, every time a medic walked past the glass-fronted room we were in, Victoria would rant at them and no one would come near us.

'I need to go to work,' she said to Mum and Dad, 'but won't leave sick niño.'

Dad thanked her and said they would take her to work and give her money to cover any loss, but he was beginning to feel that her volatile presence in the room wasn't helping. He left the room a couple of times to look for a doctor, but couldn't find one and couldn't make himself understood to any staff. At midnight, by which time I had collapsed from the pain, a doctor called Mario glided into the room. He was, according to my parents, enormous and very calm.

'Hemofílico?'

'Yes.'

'Okay,' he purred. 'Let's make life easier for him.'

Mum stood up to get the Factor VIII from the table and the doctor basically picked her up and gently placed her down on the other side of the room. He got a big thick elastic band out of his white coat and, effortlessly, swiftly, tied it round my arm, swabbed me and got the vein first time.

'You need to bring again tomorrow and I do it like that.'

The pain abated. He had flicked the switch.

We drove Victoria back to the town square and she directed us to the one bar still open. She sniffed her armpits, looked at her watch and shrugged. 'Too late,' she said.

'Too late for work?' Dad asked.

'Yes, but okay, niño come first. Niño is good.'

'Where do you work?'

'The bar.'

'Well, how much do you earn? Because we must pay you.'

'Depends who buys me a drink, maybe this much, maybe that.'

'What? Just tell me and I'll give it to you.'

'It depends.'

'On what?'

'Depends on my client.'

Mum clocked it first. Dad didn't clock it at all and kept asking until Mum leaned forward and muttered in his ear. 'She's a prostitute, Phil.'

We stopped at the cashpoint in the square and Dad paid her, possibly looking like the first client to have his wife and young child along for the, well, ride.

———

The summer drew to an end, my parents talked to me about the importance of not hiding my bleeds and then I started school.

It didn't last long.

Mum was soon called in to see the head because some parents had voiced concerns about their children being in a class with a haemophiliac and they wanted to know about HIV and the chances of catching it off me.

'What should I tell them?' the head asked.

'That they're ignorant,' Mum said. 'And so are you.'

We left soon after that.

I was moved to Elm Green Primary School. It was an independent village school where the headmistress, Mrs Mimpriss, saw things very differently. Still, some of the parents didn't want the responsibility of dealing with a haemophiliac child. There was one birthday party where every child in the class got invited except for me, because it was an activity party. I don't remember having a dramatic reaction, but I do remember feeling sad at being left out and hating the fact that I was clearly, unavoidably different.

Until then my haemophilia had been a family affair, something my parents took care of and my toddler sister was yet to understand. She got extra TV time when I was having a bleed and Mum and Dad were looking for a vein, but other than that, she was oblivious. But going to school, making friends and then not being the same as them, had brought a new element to my life, of being told 'No, you can't' – and I thought that was unfair. I hated it. I didn't want to be different. I wanted to take part. I wanted to play.

My aim was never to be a very good sportsman, all things considered. I wanted to be a very good sportsman, period. At primary school, I played football in the playground when I could, which was during those periods when one of my joints or muscles wasn't recovering from a bleed.

Everybody bleeds. But if you're not a haemophiliac, your body takes care of it without you ever knowing. When you damage a blood vessel, which is a daily occurrence, platelets clump together to block the injury. The platelets also trigger a chemical reaction to form a protective mesh made of fibrin. This chemical reaction always follows a strict pattern, with each clotting factor activated in order. That is how your body deals with bleeds. Because my liver does not produce the eighth stage in that process, Factor VIII, I keep bleeding. And it feels like breaking a bone in terms of both the pain and the debilitation.

That's why I spent many weeks of my primary school life with an arm in a sling or on crutches. There was a wheelchair parked up for me, but I never used it. I hated the sight of that thing and there was no way I was ever going to let my friends see me in it.

I wasn't bullied and teasing was rare. I was lucky. Mum and Dad found it tough when I was left out of activities and parties. They wanted the parents to say, *We want Alex there but how do we do it?* And they would have said, *We'll be there and we'll take responsibility.* But people were scared, and as an adult and now a father, I understand why. Tellingly, Mum has got friends for life from my primary school. What we experienced was a sadness that it had to be how it was, not anger or resentment. I saved that for secondary school.

Is it a cliché or an exaggeration to say that standing on the sidelines at school was the breeding ground for the determination and ability to train alone and endure the mental torture of bike racing? I've given this a lot of thought. I am the only elite athlete in the world with haemophilia. That means every other elite athlete on the planet has got there without the motivation and experience of being a bleeder. Rather than make me special, I don't think it does. It means other world-class sportsmen and women have had to find what it takes without the clear motivation I was handed. But that doesn't mean my illness hasn't shaped me. And, in the same way that haemophilia made me an outsider as a child, many of the bike riders I have known have something separate about them. Many of them are outsiders too. Putting yourself through the pain barrier in sport is not about work ethic; that's simply training hard and sticking to a diet. Pain demands an otherness, an ability to sideline yourself while you experience it because you know the potential rewards are worth it.

Every time you suffer in training or competition, you learn again that pain is temporary. It is an area on a timeline with a beginning and an end. You travel through it. The quality of your life, the levels of happiness and success available to you, are greater on the far side of that line. What the experience of my disease would gradually offer me was the insight that pain ends eventually. You can even learn to ignore it.

But if I was going to ignore my illness to any degree, we needed some guidelines. We went back to Dr Colvin.

'What can we do to help Alex's situation?' Dad asked. 'He doesn't want to be sidelined. He wants to play.'

'You have to keep him lean, keep his weight down, so his limbs don't have too much weight to carry.'

That's what Colvin said, when he could have just said, *Wrap him up in cottonwool and keep him safe.*

'Right, how do we do that?'

'Non-impact sport; swimming is ideal.'

My parents leaped on this. Within two months I was going to five different swimming lessons each week at four different pools in Essex. The local pool had only one or two lessons each week, so they took me to Maldon, Witham, Chelmsford and Colchester so that I could swim every day. Having been told there was a sport it was safe for me to do, we couldn't get enough of it.

In my last year of primary school, I joined Chelmsford Swimming Club, which was a serious club with a training regime and competitions. Mum and Dad took it in turns to get up at 5.30 a.m. to take me to the pool. Me and my club mates would bang out 50 lengths as a warm-up, then swim under instruction, and afterwards we'd go to Tesco to buy breakfast, eat it in the car, and get dropped off at school. I did that three or four times a week. The early starts were awful.

'If you wake us, we'll take you,' my parents said.

Looking back, that was genius on their part. It was their way of guaranteeing that I wasn't being forced, but I was being encouraged. I always woke them, because I wanted to go.

Mum would take a duvet and sleep in the car while I trained. I would return to the car and find her fast asleep in the half-light of a waking day. I was the sick boy told he had to sit things out, now growing stronger every morning and doing an increasingly good impersonation of a normal kid,

It was social for me too. I liked the galas. I was hanging out with people my age who hadn't seen me on crutches. I was just another boy in the pool. I went from being the slightly chubby kid who plodded round with his arms in a sling to being fit and strong. I liked swimming, but I loved being competitive. I wasn't exceptional. I made the team, but there were county standard swimmers there and I was not in their league.

It was swimming that began to turn me into an athlete. Swimming was the bedrock for what I've done since. Crawling out of bed on those early mornings, I was putting down foundations and I could not have dreamed of the career that would be built on them.

The greatest single moment of improvement in my life was the shift from reactive to preventative treatment for my disease. *Game-changing* is a colossal understatement.

Until my final year at primary school, getting a bleed would mean taking medications to fix it. That's reactive treatment. I was now moved on to prophylactic – preventative – treatment. That meant taking medication regularly, every two days, to stop bleeds occurring.

It also meant learning to inject myself.

By today's standards, I was old for this transition. There was no reversing the damage done by years of bleeds in my ankles, elbows and shoulders. These are my *target joints*, meaning a joint that has had recurrent bleeds and are now permanently damaged. I have arthritis in all of them. The way I see it, my arthritic joints are the price I paid for avoiding a near certain death sentence in the shape of HIV or Hep C infection.

I got a place at King Edward VI Grammar School in Chelmsford, known as KEGS, in 2000. I was a very lucky lad, being offered an elite education because I was naturally bright enough and had parents who nurtured that in me, as they did in my sister.

I would, on the face of it, be in a safe environment for a haemophiliac boy to mature. But sport was a big part of KEGS' identity and I was initially dismissed as irrelevant to the school's sporting life. Boys who were extremely good at sport were put on a pedestal. I observed that and felt a whole series of inarticulate but stinging feelings about it. I was a swimmer and knew I was capable, so the exclusion at KEGS angered me.

Home was the complete opposite. Mum and Dad wanted me to feel that I was good at something, that the disease wasn't going to hold me back. Sport is important in our family and that made Mum and Dad an interesting mix in that they followed the doctor's advice absolutely, but also pushed to the outer edges of what was possible. Mum credits my dad with being devoted to finding things for me to try.

Dad had a line, which came out of him, sometimes beneath his breath, as if he was thinking it all the time. Other times, he said it deliberately, looking me in the eye.

'We'll find something.'

He believed that everyone has a talent for something, but until you try things out you won't know where it lies. He was never going to settle for less for me. He saw it as his and Mum's responsibility to both protect me and Lois from harm, like all parents do, and also to protect us from a life less lived.

And I had friends who knew I was able. Tareq was the closest of them. We met early at KEGS and were often sat together because our surnames were close. I looked over his shoulder in an early French lesson and when Tareq noticed, he shifted his paper across so I could copy it more easily. Friends for life.

In my second year there, a turning point came in the shape of an inter-house multi-sports competition. It was the KEGS Olympics and my name wasn't down for anything. An older boy, the head of our house, was down for the swimming. He was very athletic; by American standards you'd call him a jock. I approached him in front of everyone and said, 'Let me take your place in the swimming.'

'Why should you?'

'Because I will win it,' I said. 'What means more to you? Your house winning or you being in the race.'

By that stage I didn't care if everyone in the room laughed at me. I already felt like an outsider and that's not a status that could get worse; you're either an outsider or you're not. I was the boy who was sent to the library while my mates were playing football, the sport I was most desperate to play. I had been offered to referee, and did it a couple of times before realising that the quickest way to become unpopular at a sporting school is to be the ref. My swimming was slightly secret because it took place outside of school. Tareq knew I swam, but few others did. The head of house didn't laugh at me or dismiss me, even though he didn't know if I could swim or not. He gave up his place to me, but with a warning.

'You'd better win it.'

I won it.

That had a huge effect on me. I was quite good at something and now everyone around me knew it.

I did some running at school and won the district race. It's not great for your joints, but as a kid you just want to run and you want to race your mates. It's on the list of things my parents might have said no to but didn't. I had a top-up of Factor VIII before I ran, leaving my levels as high as they can be, almost 100%. And off I'd go, immeasurably safer than I would have been before prophylaxis.

I wasn't a brilliant runner and I wasn't a brilliant swimmer. I could do them, but I knew I wasn't going to be world-class at either and that meant that, in time, it was an emphatic 'no' to both. They were not what I was put on this planet to do. My dad was really good at the sport he chose and it was natural for me to look at what I did in terms of *Could I be world-class?* I was a teenager, not a middle-aged man: I wasn't thinking, *What will keep me fit and healthy?* I wanted to be the best at something.

As a family, we were all thinking that I was taking Factor VIII now and not getting bleeds, *so why are we holding back?* We started to experiment with what else I could do and push things a bit. It was not without its limitations: I wasn't going to take up boxing, but dinghy sailing looked like fun and fairly safe. Dad windsurfed on the River Blackwater, and Lois and I started going along to learn dinghy sailing. I got a head injury first time out, when I took a boom to the forehead and ended up in the Royal London. To Lois' horror, the result was that we were both put in helmets after that. We were the only kids wearing them. I often wonder why Lois didn't grow up hating me.

We both liked sailing and, Dad being Dad, he put us into the winter series as well. We had seen it as a summer sport, but apparently we were wrong. That winter at the lake in Colchester we would sometimes have to break the ice to get the boats out. It was grim, but Dad doesn't do things by halves – and when that side of his personality and drive led me into tough, cold and generally less than premium situations, I found it more funny than annoying. I just loved being active and in the mix with him.

He has an obsessive nature and when he gets into a hobby or a sport, he's all in. Because he's now getting on (as I regularly remind him), he's got himself an e-bike and regularly goes to Specialized, troubleshooting issues they haven't encountered before because no one is pushing their e-bike to the extent that my dad does. It is the same side to his personality that had us out on the lake in midwinter.

I was soon cleaning up at the local sailing races, winning everything, so Mum and Dad decided I needed to go up a level and test myself.

'Let's just chuck you in the deep end find out how good you are,' Dad said, true to form.

We went to Whitstable for the last round of the National Laser Series. I liked it there. There was something about the sight of the wind farm at Herne Bay and the estuary to the west; Whitstable felt good. I had a sense that I was going to do well, until I noticed that every other sailor in my class, without exception, had new, modern white sails. Mine was slightly tatty and multicoloured. Not only did I get my arse handed to me that day, but it was very public. I stood out, you couldn't miss me. Last – but not just last, *annihilated,* and with oh such a colourful rig. I was left looking at the massive gap between me and the next level up.

It's not a long drive back to Essex from North Kent, but it was long enough to know that I didn't have what it takes to be world-class on the water. To be fair, the walk to the car from the sailing club was long enough to work that out. The sailors who had whopped me had something more than ability and strength; they had an ability to interpret the wind and feel what the boat was doing.

I didn't give up sailing immediately, but I sensed I might not have what it takes and that there was something else out there for me. And while I was still mulling all this over, my sister overtook me in a race and that was the end of it. I wasn't angry about having haemophilia, but being beaten by my baby sister out on the water? I was apoplectic.

3

FREEDOM

The Commonwealth Games, 2014

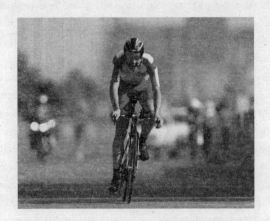

It would be too simple to call it anger, although that's in the mix. It's also to do with feeling free, riding without the weight of strategy or self-doubt on your back. Becoming a boy again on the bike. Then again, who am I kidding? Anger plays a big part. Some days, it makes me ride on another level. On occasions it has made me untouchable.

'You'd win more races if you were angrier, more selfish,' Andy Lyons said to me, mid-career, on a training ride together. 'You're not a big enough arsehole.'

Well, there's many on the World Tour who would argue with that.

I'm not an angry person. I am not that bitter person who had sand kicked in his face by life. I have been too lucky for too long to be like that. But Andy is right in some ways. There is a spark in me that gets ignited by a sense of injustice or hopelessness, and it frees me to ride at my peak. That's when I ride beyond tactics and power meters and strategy, and it feels like anger but is in fact more about removing the thought process and relying purely on instinct.

It's freedom.

But I can't access it on demand. Perhaps the great cyclists are those who can, but I'm not convinced. We're not method actors. I can't recall some previous injustice or getting dumped by a girlfriend or told I'm not allowed to play football and get an extra 20 watts out of it. Many of us on the tour suspect that Rohan Dennis *can* do this. We joke that Rohan will sit on the start line and call upon the memory of some primary school teacher saying he'd never amount to anything and turn that into a podium ride. Hats off to him if he can, because he is a superb bike rider.

It is a dangerous game, though, in professional sport, to think that mind games can make you better. Because your mind can also destroy you. The physical pain of racing can be removed by the desire to prove people wrong, but the reverse can happen too. If the pain is married to self-doubt, it can drag you down into the darkness. Perversely, you forget it all soon after a race and tell yourself, *That wasn't so bad, we'll go again tomorrow.* This self-delusion is a vital part of the toolbox. How could you get through a race as attritional as the Tour de France without it?

Alan Murchison, performance chef, mentor, friend, said to my one-time coach, Michael Hutchinson, 'Alex seems to go best when he doesn't give a shit.'

By 2014, I had been with the World Tour team Movistar for a year and had won two National TT Titles and a TT stage of the Giro. I was regarded as one of the best up-and-coming time trialists in the world. I was very happy at Movistar and about to sign another three-year contract.

At the start of each year, the team would sit down with me and take me through the race programme for the year. That year, my calendar – and my every waking thought – revolved around the UK start of the Tour de France in Yorkshire, which was to be my first Tour and the biggest moment in my career so far. Then there was the Commonwealth Games in Glasgow, which was also a massive deal for me.

Culturally, I was still making the adjustment from Team Sky to Movistar. Sky had been my first pro team and I presumed all teams worked the way they did. Movistar were very different, not lesser but less clinical. On the one hand, they had outstripped Sky in the team standings year after year and Dave Brailsford saw them as his biggest threat. On the other, once you were inside the team, their approach to their riders was laid-back to a horizontal degree, and it wasn't always clear to me what they felt strongly about and what they didn't.

The season was starting with an altitude training camp in Sierra Nevada for some of the team.

'You're going to the altitude camp,' they told me.

'Yes, sure. When is it?'

'Oh, whenever you want.'

That was kind of weird. 'Whenever I want? Okay, but who's booking my flights and accommodation?'

'You are.'

'Who's paying for this?'

'You are.'

By my standards, this wasn't a training camp but a collection of riders going to the same place under their own steam. And when they told me I would have to pay more for my accommodation than the Spanish riders, I didn't like it.

'That's not fair,' I said. 'I can go to Mallorca for free just for promoting a hotel. I'm going to do that because this isn't right. Not only should we not have to pay to go on a pre-tour training camp, but I'm not going to pay more than my teammates because I'm foreign.'

A wiser me now would just lump it and go, but I was 25 years old, on the way up and thought I knew best. I went to Mallorca, trained hard, and headed to the Tour de Suisse in great shape, but picked up a heavy cold in Switzerland and struggled.

Eusebio Unzué, the manager at Movistar, sent me a WhatsApp message in Spanish saying, 'You can't start the Tour de France if you're not healthy.' I think there was an attempt at compassion in there, but in translation it can get lost.

I rang the team. 'Sorry, mate, you were going to the Tour, but we cannot take a rider to France with a head cold, because once the Tour starts you don't get better.'

I was out. Initially, I was logical about it. I understood the decision. I knew that of all races the Tour did not carry any passengers. But soon I became distraught at missing out. To rub salt in the wounds, I had to do the pre-Tour publicity junket. Movistar were part of O2, who were one of the Tour sponsors. Going up to the O2 headquarters in Yorkshire to big up the Tour I wasn't in was hard work, but it's the sort of thing people in every career have to do; front up when behind the scenes you're raging. At one of the events, I was on a panel with the greats Nairo Quintana and Alejandro Valverde. Given their achievements and the fact that everyone at the event knew I was out of what would have been my first Tour, I felt about two inches tall. But earlier in the year, I had broken the British record for 10 miles by a large chunk and most of the questions were directed at me, simply because I was a British rider with a British record in front of a British audience.

Afterwards, Quintana and Valverde and the team were confused: 'What did you do?'

I said, 'I broke a record in the UK.'

They were nice about it, congratulated me, but totally bemused: 'Okay. Good. Well done.'

I think Movistar found me interesting because I did stuff outside of the team, which strictly speaking, in terms of my contract, I wasn't supposed to do. But those were the things they were very relaxed about. I wasn't a Spaniard and they found some of my ways, especially my love of British time trialling, quirky but acceptable. That was Movistar's way; as long as you turned up fit, they were pretty easy with what you did.

The pre-Tour press stuff ended and it was time to say goodbye to my team. I felt sick. I was very young and the disappointment of missing out on the Tour de France starting in my own backyard was more than I could handle. Stage 3, Cambridge to London, would go through my hometown of Chelmsford, the place where I was born, went to school, went to hospital a hundred times. In a Leeds car park, I watched the riders board the team bus. They headed off to join the other 21 teams in a parade in front of 10,000 people as I sat alone in my Lotus, a car that until that moment had made me feel pretty great. Valverde, our captain, saluted me and grinned through the smoked glass of the bus as it rolled past me. I tried to smile back, in an effort to send a signal of good luck and camaraderie, desperate to show I was all about the team, but my face simply looked pained.

I went home. I didn't watch the Tour. I was too furious and heartbroken. My cold cleared up on the day of the second stage and that just made me more angry. I stayed that way the whole month. I was an arsehole to be around. I took it out on everyone. My family bore the brunt. But the one thing I didn't do was get lazy. I went training. And I went hard. I hated being on the bike, hated cycling – and every day when I wanted to bail out, I dug deep and found the extra strength in the absolute fury at missing my first Tour because of a common cold.

They say a change is as good as a rest and when I could have been sitting in my room utterly depressed for a month, I was instead sitting on my bike utterly depressed for a month.

In that same pissed-off state of mind, I headed north for the Commonwealth Games, where I was competing in the road race and the time trial. The TT was an up-and-down course that left the city and cut through the countryside to the north-east of Glasgow, before returning. It suited me because it was technical, and gave the rider a lot to think about in terms of pacing and knowing where to push and where not to.

Steve Cummings was the other English competitor in the TT. I broke Steve mentally before we even started – or rather my skin suit did. Movistar were sponsored at the time by Endura. Not only were they on their way to developing one of the fastest skin suits in the world, they were also based in Scotland.

I had called them. 'Can you make me a skin suit for the Commonwealth Games? You cannot have your branding on it, but I want you to do this because I think I can do well here.'

'Yes, we can do that.'

I would tell you if it was a complex negotiation, but it wasn't. Endura jumped on board and said they believed they could help me win Gold. They didn't send me a four-page email about branding and logo opportunities to make up for the fact that the suit couldn't have their logo, they just made me the best skin suit I had ever had. When I arrived in Scotland for the Games, I went to the factory to try the suits on.

'There's actually a little bit too much material around my shoulders,' I said.

They agreed. 'We'll make you a new suit by tomorrow morning.'

Endura were so far ahead of their time. They were brilliant collaborators, especially given that one of the main problems with multi-sport events is you've got one national clothing sponsor supplying everything, rugby kits, high jump suits, swimming gear, cycling skin suits. None of those individual disciplines is their sole focus or expertise. At best they'll make everything decently; at worst it'll all be substandard. I wanted the best skin suit from the best maker and, whether out of patriotism for the Scottish Games or sheer professionalism and pride in their craft, Endura made me go faster without taking much credit for it. Their overshoes were good too.

In the dressing rooms at Glasgow, just ahead of the TT, Steve Cummings and I were together getting ready. He was putting on his kit when I took my skin suit out of my bag.

'Where d'you get that from?' he said.

'Endura. They sponsor Movistar. Said they'd make me a suit for this.'

'Is it fast?'

'Yes, it's fast.'

Steve got dressed, then wandered across to my bike. He examined it, looked over at his, then back at mine and gazed.

'It's a good bike, this Canyon, isn't it?' he said.

'Yes. It is good.'

'Fast…' he muttered.

'Yes, the Canyons are good bikes.'

'To be honest,' he said, 'I'm not super happy with this.' He nodded towards his bike.

I said, 'It looks all right.'

He took out his overshoes, flappy little Lycra things hardly worth wearing. I felt embarrassed getting mine out and I feel the same way writing about it now, because there are no euphemisms here, no macho stand-off, it was time to race and I had to get my overshoes out; the monster, bright red, perfectly fitted, superhero overshoes Endura had made for me.

Steve looked at them and just said, 'Oh, for fuck's sake.'

Nobody loves beating a teammate, but you do have to beat your teammate. If I'm first, I want him to be second, but that's as far as the goodwill goes. There was a strong field in the TT and all I knew was that, without getting on the bike, I'd already cracked Steve.

When the Commonwealths are in Europe, they're more competitive than when they are in Australia or anywhere distant from the World Tour. Riders are based in Europe and the quality of the field rises. Luke Durbridge was there, having done the Tour de France. He was my two-minute man. Michael Hutchinson was four minutes ahead of me. Geraint Thomas had come from the Tour, and he and Rohan Dennis were a lot of people's favourites.

Because of my Silver medal in the previous games, I was the second last rider to start with Dave Millar, on the brink of retirement, after me. I think Millar knew from the get-go that he wasn't going to be competitive and, sure enough, he didn't feature.

As I started, I had a vivid flashback to the car park in Leeds, after the pre-Tour de France press event, the moment where the Movistar team bus headed off for the Tour and I got into my Lotus and went home. As I did so, Eusebio drove past in his car and wound the window down and made a comment about me trying to fit my bike in the car. I know now it was a friendly attempt at a joke to a disappointed young rider for whom the wise old head of Eusebio Unzué had no words of comfort. In other words, he was just being nice. But back then, that moment felt very different. I don't know why it came into my head at the start of the TT in Glasgow and I have no recollection of the start of that ride, but there I was back in that car park and I realised that what I had felt as I sat in my shiny Lotus watching my teammates go to the Tour was not anger but humiliation. I felt small and my boss' joke had made me feel smaller, because I felt stupid owning that car when I wasn't going to the big race. That is what set me off in Glasgow, pedalling like a maniac with a snarl in my ride.

FUCK THAT SHIT.

And I flew, like someone had poured acid on my arse.

Paul Manning was in the car giving me radio feedback. I was fastest at the first checkpoint, fastest at the second checkpoint. It was a great crowd in Glasgow.

This was the first Games since the London Olympics two years earlier and a similar energy was now radiating from the crowds lining the route. I rode so hard, so physically and with so much attitude, that thinking and pain dissolved. I caught Michael Hutchinson, my idol as a kid and the guy that I hoped, and my Dad hoped, I'd be as good as one day. Then I caught Luke Durbridge, obliterated from his first Tour de France.

The only problem with riding like that and trying to describe it now is that it was a blur. A big, angry, beautiful, just about perfect blur. But not perfect because Paul Manning's voice told me I'd slipped to second fastest at the third checkpoint and slipped down to third fastest at the fourth. Geraint Thomas and Rohan Dennis were both ahead of me.

FUCK THIS.

I went crazy. Super-disciplined, perfect technique, outwardly calm, inwardly crazy. I powered like I was just starting. We came into the park section in Glasgow, which was full of corners. There was a drain on one corner. Generally, you avoid them because they're more slippery than tarmac. I intended to avoid it but made a late decision to take the fastest line possible.

I'd rather crash than come second.

That's where I won it.

I finished and the Team England crew at the line rushed up to me. 'You're first.'

'Are you sure? Are you sure? Because last time I heard Rohan and Geraint were up on me.'

'You're first.'

Millar was more than two minutes off me. We didn't need to wait for him to finish. I had beaten two of the best time trialists of the era and both came across immediately to shake hands with me. Rohan was friendly. Geraint was his usual dry self.

'I've just come from the Tour. I'm tired. I'm on my hands and knees. That was the speed I had today. I couldn't go any faster, but I could have done another two or three laps.'

Typical Geraint. Pragmatic about his ride, totally friendly, but convinced he had lost the race and that's why I'd won it. Three days later he won the road race. He was happy. He even smiled at one point.

I'm good friends with Rohan and he was generous to me about the win, even seemed happy for me. But backstage, behind the podium, as we got ready to go up for the presentation an over-officious member of the Games team insisted he cover up a logo on his socks and Rohan lashed out with a verbal tirade. Geraint and I looked at each other. Angry Rohan; generous in defeat but at the same time raging with anger at having had Gold snatched from him right at the end.

In the nine years since that day, the following dialogue occurs between us every time we see each other.

'Hey, Rohan, remember Glasgow?'

'Hey, Alex, was that the last time you ever beat me?'

The podium was one of those pinch-me moments because it was on Glasgow Green, the main park in Glasgow, on a large music festival stage with a massive audience. My parents were there, my auntie and Sky Andrew. My name blared out, a Gold medal was hung around my neck, 'Jerusalem' was sung as the flag of St George went up. It was spine-tingling.

I didn't plan my interviews and the next day when I read the papers I was surprised by what I'd said. A lot of British athletes other than me had medalled that day. Tom Daley had, I think, won Silver. Every winner's interview read the same. *Really happy, worked hard for this, this medal has been my dream. Thanks to my coach. Thanks to my mum and dad. Thanks to my husband/wife.*

Mine wasn't like that.

'I have spent this last month so angry,' I said in one.

I hadn't intended to say any of it. But it poured out. I don't remember most of what I said, but James Riach in the *Guardian* reported it like this:

> It should have been a glorious moment for Alex Dowsett, riding through his home county during the third stage of this year's Tour de France. Yet with people lining the streets to celebrate, one man was hurting, vexed with rage and drowning in disappointment while he watched from the sidelines. Yet, without that pain, without that devastation, Thursday's victory on the roads of Scotland would not have been possible. It was, he conceded, a display motivated by anger, emotion coursing through his veins as much as the

adrenalin that dragged him over the line after a brutal 47 minutes. The Essex
boy who turned up to last week's England media briefing in a pair of maroon
loafers departed Glasgow Green feeling like he had diamonds on the soles of
his shoes.

It has always been this way since I started cycling competitively as a teenager. I usually pull something significant out of the bag when I'm angry and then go and apologise to the people who have had to live with me. That kind of anger is not wild or dramatic. It is made of steel and is very intense. It is locked away in the part of me that coils up in self-defence at having been born diseased and jabbed a few hundred times with a needle when too young to understand why. It sometimes explodes, unleashes the fear and frustration, and that's when I am free.

Movistar really didn't understand the Commonwealth Games. I get that. Explaining the Commonwealth in the modern day is not a walk in the park. But they saw there was a huge amount of press around my Gold and they messaged me.

'Alex, what have you won? What is this? It seems to be big.'

I gave a *Commonwealth Games For Dummies* explanation.

'Cool, Alex. Well done. Now come back to work.'

And I did. As Commonwealth Champion. And in a better mood.

4

ONE EVENING, ON THE RIVER BLACKWATER

The Beginning, 2001

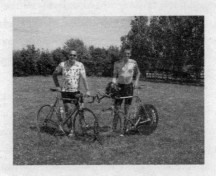

My dad would windsurf a local spot called St Lawrence Bay on the River Blackwater. It's moody and exposed, sometimes bleak, often beautiful, miles of mudflats, creeks and inlets peppered with abandoned boats, in the shadow of the decommissioned nuclear power station at Bradwell. South-westerly winds race unopposed across the flat farmland and marshes of the Dengie peninsula and Dad would meet them on an incoming tide, bombing out across the flat shallow waters between Osea Island and the shore. If you get into trouble there, the next stop is the North Sea.

One autumn evening in 2001 he was out on the water, looked upriver and saw windsurfers going faster than he was, across Maylandsea Bay. He decided he wanted some of that action, so he got in the van and chased the wind. He met a bunch of guys up there and one of them was called Eric Smith. Dad and Eric windsurfed together that evening, in a monster breeze, with the currents ripping out at nine knots. Afterwards, as they de-rigged, they got chatting. Eric was into racing bikes and so was his son. Dad said it sounded interesting.

'Is your boy any good?' Dad asked.

'He's pretty good,' Eric said. 'There's two of them showing promise, my son Glen and a lad called Mark Cavendish.'

Now, my dad's midlife crisis took many forms and one of them was mountain biking. (To be fair to him, he is still doing it 20 years later.) Eric Smith joined him on his Thursday night mountain biking sessions in the woods up on Danbury ridge, the highest point in Essex. It was near to where we lived and I started going along too. I wasn't supposed to, it wasn't on the list of safe sports and we were straying from the security of the swimming pool – but I was with Dad, which always felt safe, and I was still searching for something. On the undulating mud tracks of Danbury Woods, under the canopy of ancient oaks and towering pines, I thought I might be finding it.

Cycling shares with swimming the quality of being good as a non-impact sport. And that's where the similarities end because cycling is only a non-impact sport until you crash. At which point it becomes a terrible idea.

I went mountain biking in a small group every weekend. Tareq joined in. He'd get a lift up to my parents and come with myself and Shaun Hurrell (who went on to represent Team GB in mountain biking). After the ride we'd go back to my house, where Tareq lived for Mum's honey barbequed sausages. If she was out or busy, he'd get tomato soup and a cup of tea from me. Still does.

Dad and I went out for a ride together one Sunday and he took me up a 1.5km, 5% climb on Danbury Hill. I powered up it, pushing myself for the first time into a horrible, dark place on the bike. I had no idea why I had done it, why I hadn't eased off so that it hurt less. It had happened instinctively. When Dad arrived at the top, I was throwing up. But I was not in the slightest way bothered. What was happening to me physically was of no interest. It was what I had done to myself mentally that meant something. The place I had just driven myself to psychologically shocked me. I could not stop thinking about it, a place in my head where I was utterly alone and untouchable, enduring physical discomfort that was not entirely new, but withstanding a level of mental torture that was. And at the same time it was a choice I had made, something I bore because I could. Not because I had to, but because I could.

Dad had been around elite sportspeople for years and, although the ones he knew and could count himself among strapped themselves to engines, the mentality was recognisable. I had crossed a threshold that afternoon. Not only had I found myself able to push myself to new levels physically and psychologically, but I had come out the other side with a hunger for more. Soon, I lived for Thursday night mountain biking with Dad and his mates. I'd come back covered in mud and grinning like an idiot.

Eric Smith never missed a Thursday either and he invited us all to spend a Bank Holiday Monday at their house in Battlesbridge, where I fell in love for the first time.

The object of my desire was a red, aluminium Eddy Merckx road bike that belonged to Eric. I stood and stared: traditional Columbus tubing, a Rolls saddle, Campagnolo Chorus Groupset, Campag flat profile rims, and the blue Michelin tyres that were fashionable at the time and transformed my eyeballs into red thumping hearts. I couldn't believe a bike could look this cool. And I couldn't help myself.

Well, I did help myself.

Mum and Dad were chatting with Jan Smith when Eric appeared and said, 'Your son just nicked my bike.'

Yup. That road bike just called to me and I was off, having lowered the seat, taking it for a test drive. It was uncharacteristic of me: I was a polite boy and fairly shy, but I had no control over myself from the moment I saw the bike. Riding out on it, I felt I belonged to a bike this good. Together, we ate up the road with the breathlike sound that a perfectly set-up bike has. It was the first time I had heard it. I was too absorbed by the synergy of my body, brain and the bike to think about the fact I had taken it without asking or to dwell on the reaction I would get on my return.

When I did get back, the adults were standing in the driveway waiting for me, looking concerned but not angry. I realised as I swung in that they were looking at the bike, not me – and once they could tell that the bike was unharmed, they relaxed.

I got off the bike and wheeled it across to Eric, fully intending to apologise. Even as I opened my mouth, I thought I was going to say sorry. But I didn't.

I said: 'Dad, I love that bike so much.'

Mum said, later, that I sounded possessed.

The adults laughed. Eric took the bike from me and rested his hand on my shoulder, and I felt the small pat of his hand that told me he didn't mind. He liked me. And I was lucky that he did because Eric Smith knew cycling inside out and he took me under his wing. He immediately moved me to a fixed gear bike because he wanted me to learn how to deal with changes in incline by adapting my pedalling speed rather than by using the gears.

I would ride with Glen, Eric's son, whom I idolised. He and Cavendish raced for a team called Dataphonics. Eric and Glen put me into my local time trial race, the Maldon 10, and I clocked 28:01. I was quick straight away because I was fit from thousands of hours in the pool. Swimming had taught me to regulate my breathing and cycling demanded the same skill. The downside was my broad swimmer's shoulders, which for cycling, and time trialling especially, are the last thing you want. Many hours of my professional life have been devoted to finding a grip on the handlebars and a tuck position that best alleviates the aerodynamic losses of my shoulders.

There was a hurdle to overcome. It was time to update Dr Colvin on the direction my sporting life was going in and to get his guidance. We didn't know how he would react and went into see him at the Royal London with a degree of nervousness.

'It looks like road bike racing is going to be a thing,' Dad said.

There isn't any tumbleweed in Whitechapel, but if there were, some would have rolled across the consultation room at this point. Dr Colvin looked at me doubtfully, maintaining eye contact longer than usual or comfortable. He bowed his head and pressed the fingers of both hands together and stared at them for what felt like forever.

'We'd rather you played chess,' he said.

My heart sank. He looked up at my parents, then at me, right at me, and his very modest, unassuming smile appeared.

'But if that's what you want to do, we will support you.'

Not long after that, Dad was down at Maldon CC with me when he was taken aside by the club secretary, Dave Tyas.

'Your son's very good,' Dave said.

Dad shrugged it off. 'Yes, he seems to be doing okay.'

'No. You don't understand. Your son is very good.'

'Well, how do you know? He's just a kid on a bike.'

Dad knew cars but nothing about bike racing, none of us did.

'No,' Dave said, 'he's not just a boy on a bike, you can tell; his legs move, his body doesn't. That is the natural talent in any of these top people and he's got it. We're putting him in the GHS. His Maldon 10 time will qualify him.'

'What's the GHS?'

'The George Herbert Stancer Memorial – it's the National Youth Time Trial Championship.'

Dad was gobsmacked. Eric Smith said to him, 'He needs a good bike, Phil, and it's going be a couple of grand.'

'Do you think he's worth it? Is Dave right about Alex?'

'Yes.'

Eric then introduced us to Steve China. Eric and Glen felt they'd done everything for me that they could and that Steve was now the guy to take me forward. He had won a lot of races as a cyclist in Essex, raced cars and is an engineer.

Eric said to me, 'Go with Steve. He's a perfectionist.'

At the time Steve was developing a bike with Eddy Merckx and he sold it to us. He was straightforward right from the off.

'Be there at 9. A minute past 9, I'm gone.'

Once we started riding, it was a similar story.

'When I change gear, you change gear. When I drink, you drink; when I stop for a pee, you stop for a pee. Let's go, don't fall off the back of my wheel.'

Then he'd tear off and keeping up with him would leave me ruined. I was 14. After one of the early ride-outs, Steve and I finished back at our house and my dad asked him how I'd done.

Steve nodded and said, 'A little bit of talent, a very good work ethic. He could do something.'

Everything we learned, we got from Steve. I would not have had my career if he had not come into our lives at the exact moment he did. A brilliant mind and generous, he'd help anybody that showed promise. But if you turned up late or ate badly, he'd tell you to go home.

I started cycling to school. The deputy head teacher at KEGS was called Mr Bevan and the most visible thing to us about him was that he cycled too. And he looked quite serious about it. It turned out he was cycling 20 miles each way to KEGS and competing for Cambridge University in time trials, but none of us knew that. Cycling had not yet had the mass explosion in popularity which would see British Cycling's membership double between 2008 and 2012. So, Mr Bevan was an oddity. Even fellow staff members took the piss out of him.

From Year 9 onwards I was taught maths by Mr Bevan and we'd chat a bit about cycling. There weren't many pupils cycling to school, the bike sheds were knackered and I had this stupidly valuable bike. We all used to see Mr Bevan wheel his bike into his office in the morning and I asked if I could keep my bike in his office too.

He looked at my bike and raised an eyebrow. 'Yeah, you better had.'

I would have a quick chat about cycling and what I was up to when I dropped my bike off. He listened and encouraged me without putting pressure on me. He never questioned its safety and I never talked about my haemophilia. He was one of the very few people I told about going to compete in the GHS.

It was a day trip from Essex up to Staffordshire. Early starts were not an issue to me, I had been doing them for years, but that morning the familiar lanes and streets around our home in Great Baddow looked different. Nervous anticipation coursed through me. Eric Smith and his wife Jan came with us, which was handy because Dad and I didn't have a clue how a serious bike race worked.

The GHS National TT championship was aimed at discovering the best up-and-coming time trialists. There was a field of 120 riders, and from the moment we arrived, it was clear that I was at the very young and inexperienced end of the scale, with plenty of muscular 16-year-olds towering over me. I went off early as one of the slowest qualifiers. My Personal Best for 10 miles at that point was around 23 minutes. The field went off at one-minute intervals, so when I finished there was the best part of 2 hours to wait.

I did 21 minutes, 12 seconds and punctured after the finish, so I had a long walk back to the HQ. I passed a group of people drinking outside a pub. Some of them noticed me and smiled or laughed, which I thought was strange until I saw it from their point of view: here was a little kid in a skin suit with a pointy helmet and bare feet walking up the high street.

I stopped and looked at my reflection in a shop window. I looked like a cyclist. My bike looked as cool as Eric Smith's. This was a National Youth Time Trial and I had completed it. I didn't have a clue how well how I had done, but I was here, doing it.

In your mid teens you start doing things in your own right and it dawns on you slowly that this is your own life and personality you are beginning to inhabit. You are changing from being someone's kid into your own unique self. My life was changing. In some ways, it was starting. And as I got back to the start area and looked for Dad, it changed again because my name was at the top of the leader board.

I was the fastest time by a large margin – and for the first of what would be many times in my life, I waited to see who would go faster. One by one the riders came in, all slower than me. My name stayed at the top of the board and I hardly took my eyes off it. Dad presumed my lead was down to me going off early and not being the worst rider there. But with 60 riders still to go, Eric turned to me and said, 'You could win this.'

A hunger – a tingling, disbelieving, panic-stricken desire – shot through me. Suddenly, I wanted this more than I had ever wanted something in my life.

I heard Dad mutter to Eric, 'You serious?'

Eric nodded. 'I can't believe it,' he said. 'He could, and no one's heard of the kid.'

And so we waited and all the time we waited I stared at my own name at the top of the leader board. It still looked like a foreign object. And with just one rider left to start, my name was still there.

The last boy to ride that day was another Essex-born teenager, Ian Stannard. He was two years older, much bigger, a fully developed young man with stubble – a monster. As he set off, I was already being notified that I had won the 14-year-old and 15-year-old categories. And then, at the halfway mark in Ian's ride, I was ahead by four seconds. The day was becoming more and more unbelievable by the minute. Dad was getting excited. My thoughts were not fully formed enough for me to feel anything. I was in shock.

Ian told us subsequently that when trailing me by 4 seconds at the halfway split, someone screamed at him, 'You're 10 seconds down to some little kid,' and he wrecked himself to win it. He came in at 20.59, 13 seconds ahead of me, a worthy winner. I watched the scoreboard as my name slipped to second and Ian's appeared at the top.

And I felt . . . fantastic.

I had come second in my first serious race and in a field where everyone else in the top 10 was 16 years old.

This is it, I thought, *this is the sport I'm good at.*

That's when I fell in love with cycling.

We'll find something, boy.

We had found it. Very soon I would turn into a boy and then a young man who could get distraught at coming second. Not that day, though. That day was one of the greatest days of my life and second was absolutely beautiful. I could not have imagined then that Ian Stannard and I would go on to be teammates together at Team Sky and Team GB, and close friends.

In the following two years, 2004 and 2005, I would win this race, but my second place in 2003 was way more important and far more precious. That was the start. I took a last look at my name on the leader board and I remembered something Dad had said to me once: that there's a Michael Schumacher-level talent of racing driver walking up and down Chelmsford high street, but until the opportunity comes, it'll never be realised.

On the way home, I threw up from exhaustion and Jan Smith said to Dad, 'It's a really good thing he's throwing up because it means he can push himself.'

'Yeah,' Dad said, 'I already knew that about him.'

Would I have even started time trial racing if people like Steve China and the Smiths hadn't helped me, pushed me, given me their time and knowledge, and been honest about the discipline and effort needed to get anywhere? Not a chance.

I remember the drive back from Staffordshire more vividly than I do the race itself. How many times had my dad had to pile me into a car as I lay in my mother's arms crying while somewhere inside my body I bled? How miserable and scared had he felt driving me to hospital countless times? And now, here we both were, and I was a fit and strong 14-year-old who could not wipe the grin off my face. I had never felt so happy. I was buzzing. I could not wait to get home and tell Mum and Lois all about it. I could not wait to get back on my bike.

I looked at Dad, at his face in profile as he drove us home, the little grin. The fact that he had been so good at his sport had always been there in the background of my life, and it fed a natural desire to want to be good at something too. Today I felt I had found my version of Dad's motor racing. I was proud that he was a member of the British Racing Drivers' Club, an elite club he was invited to join after he got the Silver Star Award in 1988 for the best British-based British car racer. I remember the day I saw his name on the wall at Silverstone and hearing stories that his colleagues would tell me about just how good he was, because he had raced in an era when you had to be either very talented or very rich, and he was certainly not the latter.

Dad has always been humble about his career. He'd tell stories of how a race was won or funny anecdotes about the trials and tribulations of his racing life, but he never told me how good he was. I know from looking it up that he had a staggering record of making the podium in 53% of his 112 races, but he never told me. He did have a trophy cabinet, but it was tucked away, out of sight. Lois and I would go to it and play with the trophies and make up our own awards ceremonies.

———

It is two decades since that euphoric second place at the GHS and our drive home to Essex. Very soon I will return from living abroad to living in the Essex countryside. I intend to take a ride up to Marylandsea Bay and have a look out over the water because that is where this all started. That evening on the River Blackwater, if Dad hadn't got in the van and gone in search of stronger winds, if he'd settled for less of a ride or packed up and gone home, if he hadn't been looking for the biggest buzz and physical challenge he could find, then he wouldn't have met Eric Smith and I wouldn't have had Glen Smith to emulate.

It is sometimes miraculous how one moment can shape your life. It can also be terrifying to think how easily it might not have happened.

Windsurfers have a saying, *Go big or go home*. When sizing up the wind strength and deliberating what sail to use, it's better to have too much power than too little; it's more fun too. Dad could have stayed in the lighter winds that evening on the Blackwater but he saw other sailors bombing across the bay and he wanted a taste of it. He came in, de-rigged, drove in his soaking wetsuit upriver and rigged up again, to push himself and have more fun. That's the approach to life that he and Mum gave me. We'll tread our own path. We'll find something. We'll live with haemophilia in our own way. And we'll go big.

5

THE HUNGER GAMES

The British Academy, 2007–2009

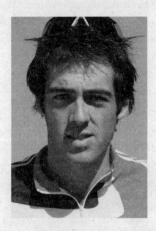

Robin Bevan, my maths teacher at KEGS, did not look like an athlete or an inspiration. He looked exactly like a maths teacher. Neat, compact, bespectacled. But he was an exceptional cyclist, had a steely resolve and focus to him, believed strongly in justice and fairness, was President of the National Education Union, and changed my life.

He couldn't get me to like maths – he was only human, after all – but as well as letting me park my Carrera bike in his office, Mr Bevan sent me into a tailspin of nervous excitement by arranging for the Olympic talent team to visit our school. It was, for some weeks, the only thing on my mind. On the day, the team from British Cycling put the 20 pupils who had signed up through a straight-line sprint course and then a longer sustained ride which was used to observe us for pedal cadence, bike position and what they saw as pace potential. They timed the long ride and I posted one of the fastest times in the country. Dave Nichols, who now leads the cycling development squads at Loughborough University, was picked up through that talent team, and so were Shaun Hurrell and me.

'You're raising eyebrows,' Mr Bevan said to us.

I liked the sound of that.

The dream scenario from this point on was leaving school to go to the Academy, the Under-23 Great Britain cycling team. As that dream took on the air of plausibility, Dad got worried. Somewhere along the line, his and Mum's ambition for me not to spend my life in a wheelchair and to get a good education leading to a nice, safe, decently paid job, had morphed into my ambition to be a professional cyclist, which meant both a constant physical danger and no further education. That had never been the plan.

Dad and Mr Bevan had a conversation about my future and my efforts to balance training, racing and schoolwork. I was doing well enough in my studies, but it was clear that my mind was on cycling, not academia. Dad knew from personal experience that you get only one chance at a sports career, so one of his questions was whether I was good enough to risk my education for it.

There are not many teachers who have the vision and bravery to tell a parent not to worry about their child's education.

'Alex can complete his A levels,' he said. 'He can go off and ride with the Academy. It's not the end of the world if it doesn't work out. Any university will be glad to have him after the Academy if that's how it turns out.'

Meanwhile, I was struggling with the idea that taking my A levels seriously meant not getting to be a pro cyclist. I know, it sounds like the mother of all excuses, the thinking athlete's version of *the dog ate my homework*, but for me it was a real concern that the backup of an education meant I wasn't committed to the bike, when all I really cared about was succeeding on the bike. This was an attitude that could have led to a disastrous showing in my exams, but I was lucky; the Academy came in for me early and we negotiated a deal that meant I would spend the first half of 2007 racing U23 in the UK and studying for my A levels, and then the moment I finished school I would join the U23 GB cycling team in Italy for the second half of their season.

The Academy was the brainchild of Rod Ellingworth, an affable, tough, Lancastrian rider turned coach with a work ethic and attention to detail that surpasses anyone who has trained me. Some of the finest cyclists to ever wear a Team GB skin suit consider him a mentor. Mark Cavendish described him perfectly when he said that Rod never got angry, but the thought of disappointing him was terrifying. Rod's standards are impeccable.

The Academy has been responsible for 90% of the British professionals in the peloton now. It was designed to break you. If you didn't survive the Academy, you were finished. If you did, you might not be. It was a dream factory, run on hope and designed to destroy your ambition to become a pro unless you were exceptional. The working conditions were, at times, Victorian. The winter was spent in Manchester, training on the track and on the road, in a boot camp. For the summer, you moved to Tuscany, which might sound idyllic, but only if your idea of a good time was eight or nine young men living under the same roof with the same dream, eating, drinking, sleeping and training together, and trying to smash each other into cycling oblivion on the road.

Let's just say, the dynamic was complex.

And I didn't get off to the best of starts. Having joined up halfway through the year, in Italy, and with that stigma of the pupil who had joined school after everyone else had become friends, I kicked off my first boot camp winter in Manchester by oversleeping on my first day.

The moment I woke up, I knew something was wrong. The room, which was spartan at the best of times, and the corridors outside, were too quiet and I could sense that I was too alone in this building for it to be right. I grabbed my phone. It was dead. By the time I got the charger in and switched it back on, it was five to eight. My stomach flipped.

'No, no, no, no!'

My phone battery had been playing up for a while, and during the night it had died and my alarm hadn't gone off. I was late for our very first track session. We were meant to be at the track at seven, ready to start at eight. I rang Rod at three minutes to.

'I'm so sorry, my phone died in the night. I'm having problems with it. I guess that it's not worth me coming in for this session, but I will, of course, if you want me to. I'm so sorry. I'll be there for this afternoon session.'

'No, you won't,' he said, and hung up.

I was terrified. And massively hacked off because I was never late for anything. Early starts were my bread and butter.

Once I was dressed, I sat in my room and waited, catastrophising for Britain. *I'll be kicked out. No uni will want me. I'm flipping burgers.*

When the morning session ended, Rod called me. 'You're coming to the track. You've got some cars to clean.'

I was relieved he was still talking to me.

Rod was waiting for me – and monosyllabic. He pointed to the bucket, sponge and the tap, and he showed me the exact cars he wanted cleaned. I didn't say much, not being a total idiot, and got stuck in. After 10 minutes, a car drew into the car park and parked as close to the athlete's entrance as possible. Chris Hoy got out. I straightened up and watched as I took in the geography of my situation; anyone entering for afternoon practice was going to walk past me, which Chris Hoy then did, with a barely concealed grin.

It was deliberate. I spent the afternoon washing cars in exactly the spot where everyone on the GB squad would get a good look at the young kid getting punished on the first day of boot camp. Vicky Pendleton laughed knowingly as she saw me. She probably knew it was Rod's way.

Maybe the same thing happened to her, I told myself, without believing it.

Jason Queally rocked up. Seeing him win Gold in Athens as an eight-year-old was one of my earliest memories, not because I was into cycling but because he started appearing on my cereal boxes soon afterwards.

That afternoon, I bought myself an alarm clock. I was never late for another session in my life. I was horrified that Rod now perceived me as *that guy* – and with every reason. I struggled in my early career worrying about what people thought. I suffered huge anxiety. As I've got older, it's something that I have learned to master. I've conducted myself in a way I consider proper, pushed for high standards from my teams, said something about riders who behave badly and gradually learned not to care so much about what people who don't know me think of me.

But in the Academy, I was nowhere near being able to do those things. I was mature in some ways, in that I was disciplined (failed alarm calls notwithstanding), hard-working and more than capable of putting myself through pain and pressure. But I had also been looked after and overprotected, and was lazy in certain regards.

In Italy, we had to share a bedroom with one other rider. In Manchester, we lived in flats, two people per flat enjoying the luxury of their own bedroom. Manchester was easier than Italy: although you couldn't go home, you could go out. Saturday nights were a no-go because the coaches always made us do a monster ride out into the Peak District on a Sunday. But we took other opportunities when they arose. We lived in Fallowfield, which was Student Central, so we were surrounded by temptation. We were in a block of flats with the mountain bikers, the BMXers, male and female squads.

There was an unusual dynamic in that we all went through a lot together – the training, having no cash, the losing out on a young adult's social life for the chance of a pro career, and the dog-eat-dog backdrop to our existence together – and that was a bond of sorts. But, at the same time, we were not mates.

We tolerated each other while striving for the same goal, knowing few of us would get it. I found it an achingly lonely experience. There wasn't a single day I did not speak to either Mum or Dad. I would not have coped otherwise.

Years later, as riders in the World Tour, I would happily chat in the bunch with guys from the Academy. Back then, amid the tensions and darker undertones, there were only two people I considered friends: Russell Hampton, an outstanding road racer that I always look forward to seeing when we meet up in Essex, and Andy Tennant, a man who overcame a heart condition to win 15 Gold medals in individual and team pursuit events, including being in the Great Britain pursuit team that won Gold at the World Championships in Melbourne. Andy was a dear friend throughout the Academy and I was best man at his wedding.

But having those two men to trust and talk to did not come close to making the Academy comparable to the university experience some of my friends were having. If eight students were put in a house together and told there were two degrees up for grabs between them, and about four units of alcohol per week per head, then you might get close.

At the Academy you were fighting against each other for places in the team, you were fighting against each other to be the protected rider in a race – and if you lost that fight, your role became to fetch bottles for your competitors. Everyone was looking to get an angle or get one over on you, to psychologically break you down. That was part of the game. And sometimes, the game became toxic.

One evening in my second year, when I was flat-sharing in Manchester, I'd gone out on a date. When I got back, I thought we'd been burgled. My bedroom had been annihilated; the bathroom was in a disgusting state. But then I saw that Ben's room hadn't been touched and I realised that nothing of mine had been stolen, although my food had been half eaten and discarded. I began to shake and a hot, stinging sensation moved down my spine. At first, it was disbelief, as I processed what the carnage around me – total destruction but no theft – meant. After a few minutes standing amid the wreckage, not sure whether I felt angry or scared, I settled for feeling monumentally pissed off while deciding I would put the room straight, never mention it, train like a legend and not give whoever had done this the satisfaction of a reaction.

I'm going to work and win and get a pro contract and never look back.

But then I discovered my wash bag was soaked in urine and my bed had been pissed on. They had written obscenities about my mum on the whiteboard. Now, I was raging. But I cleaned up the room and kept my mouth shut.

I knew my dad would drive from Essex to Manchester in an instant to take me home if I asked. There was not a cell in my body that didn't want to ask, but I knew that would be my cycling career over. All that night, I fought the urge to call home the way I imagine an alcoholic resists reaching for the bottle. At times, I had Dad's number up, my finger fractionally above the screen. I played on a continuous loop in my head what would happen to my career and me if I left and went home, admitted weakness, gave up. None of the possible scenarios saw me ever riding a bike for a pro team or for my country. And I thought about the effect on whoever had done this to me if they saw me stronger, saw me training harder, saw me getting better than them and not giving a monkey's. I liked that. I focused on that, knowing I was right not to call home and at the same time desperately wanting to.

I'm stronger than you, whoever you are.

I said nothing to the others. I behaved as normal, hid my anger and fear, but made no effort to appear especially buoyant. I observed everyone around me, said nothing but allowed the space and opportunity for the truth to come out. A few days later, two of my teammates, who had not been involved in the trashing, told me what had happened; there had been one ringleader who had done the damage and two others who went with him and didn't do anything, but also did nothing to stop it happening.

I had always wondered if my face didn't fit at the Academy, maybe a north–south thing, maybe I was perceived as educated and therefore posh (although having an A level in woodwork wasn't a hanging offence last time I looked), but listening to the other guys I accepted that it was more down to one person being a colossal arsehole and disliking me, rather than anything more deep-rooted or widely felt. I never said anything about it to Rod or my folks. And I lived with the feeling of humiliation it had left. Erasing that was part of a long-term plan called turning pro.

A few weeks later Mum, Dad and Lois came up to Manchester for a weekend. *Christ! It was good to see them.* We had a great time and it was just what I needed, but it made saying goodbye to them incredibly hard.

Too hard, it turned out.

We went out for dinner. We laughed a lot. We didn't talk about cycling. We talked about everything but, I made sure of that. Lois and I took the piss out of each other and loved every second of it. As the meal went on, I felt my insides begin to tighten at the thought of them leaving and heading back to Essex, and me returning to my digs.

Dad drove us back to Fallowfield and we all got out of the car outside my building. I gave Lois a big hug and Mum an even bigger one, and I held her tight for a moment longer than I might have done.

'You okay?' she whispered.

'Yeah.'

I made sure I had a nice big smile on my face for her when she looked. As Dad gave me a hug and a slap on the back, I broke down. For a moment I thought my legs were going to give way beneath me. I started crying.

'I'm alright,' I said and attempted some sort of a smile. A smile that was undermined by the fact I was sobbing.

Dad drew me back in to him. He held me tight and whispered, 'Tell me.'

The truth came out. Every detail. I'll never forget the look of disbelief on my parents' faces and the sheer rage on my sister's. I told them a dozen times I didn't want them to say or do anything about it. They humoured me by agreeing, kept a lid on their outrage in front of me, and as soon as they got home to Essex they called Rod Ellingworth, at one o'clock in the morning, and they let him have it with both barrels.

By this time, the guys involved were out in Italy, racing. Rod Ellingworth put down the phone to my parents and immediately called Max Sciandri, the new director of the Academy, and ordered him to put the riders on the first plane home. They were kicked out for a month.

I know it's not cool for a fully grown man to have his mum and dad standing up for him. You might think I shouldn't have told them, but I simply do not have that relationship with my parents. We share our stuff. That's what *family* is for us. We look after each other. People can call that babyish if they like, I couldn't care less. I was 19 years old. The parents of one of the riders involved went to my parents and complained that their son had been the victim of the incident, had taken the brunt and was hardly guilty. Fifteen years on, just thinking about Mum's response still makes me laugh. To be polite, I could say she disavowed them of that notion. In reality, she tore them a new one.

We are all different people now. Not only have I grown up – and I needed to – but a lot of the riders who made life unpleasant for me back then are different human beings now. Some of them I've known for a long time in the peloton and I like them. We were worlds apart at the time, but we've matured together professionally.

For a long time after the incident and the fallout, I lived on edge and was sometimes close to breaking point. If I did go out for the evening or have a weekend back home, I'd return wondering what was waiting for me.

One evening a couple of months later, Dad dropped me off in Manchester. I didn't want to be back in Manchester or at the Academy, but I tried to hide it. We'd had a great weekend back home and Dad had driven me back not because I needed or expected him to, but because we both loved the time on the road together. There had been no further incidents, but I lived in constant fear of reprisal, of another incident, of some small token of the same hatred that seemed to have gone into violating my space the first time. Every time I returned to the flat and let myself into my bedroom, I would sweat from the spike in cortisol levels.

I had said nothing to hint at any of this, but I was very quiet as Dad and I got close to Manchester that night. When it came to saying goodbye, Dad wrapped his arms around me and whispered, 'Alex, you don't have to stay here. I can take you home.'

I whispered back, 'I want to stay.'

I can't think of many times I've lied to my dad, but that was one of them.

Italy was regarded as the hardest and most competitive U23 race calendar in the world. That's why we spent the summers training and racing there. If you won a race in Italy, you went pro. If you won a race in the UK, nobody batted an eyelid.

We were based in Quarrata in Tuscany. When I first got there, Rod sat me down and said, 'You've missed half the year, so there's zero pressure on you. It doesn't matter if you only last 60km of a race, or even 40. None of that matters. There's no pressure at all.'

I was confused. I said to him, 'Lasting the race? I've been riding against fully grown men in the UK and coming top 10 most of the time. This is Under-23s, I'm going to be winning these races.'

I lasted 60km in my first race in Italy, took an absolute belting and got shelled out the back. Rod was spot on. I did not finish a race in Italy for the rest of that year. In the next three years, my best result in Italy was a seventh place on a day when the weather was so appalling that only 11 riders out of 180 finished.

There was a lot going on in the Italian U23 scene back then, but that did not include drug testing. There was none of that. It was like the Wild West. Some perspective: the first half of 2007 when I was still at school, I was winning National Bs in men's races in the UK. I won the Perfs Pedal race. I had a lot of success and was only a part-time athlete. Italian riders regularly winning in Italy at Under-23 level would then turn pro, where there is testing, and take an absolute kicking. Similarly, at U23 I couldn't live with them on climbs and then, in the pro ranks, suddenly I was a better climber than them. They would last a couple of years and then lose their contracts.

You never went into races with the mentality that you were up against riders who were taking drugs, but the way the Italian U23 scene worked you'd have to be deluded not to put the pieces together. We all experienced it, seeing a rider roll up to the start line with bloodshot eyes and win the race with ease while Academy riders like Peter Kennaugh, Andy Tennant and myself, who have all gone to win races as pros, were way off the pace.

Italy was a breathtakingly lonely experience. There was nowhere to go and you were often rooming with someone you wouldn't choose as a mate. I was broke, living off 60 quid a month, while my mates back home were enjoying the best years of their young life at uni or earning money. On rare breaks back home I'd go on tour, to a couple of friends at uni in York and Leeds, and to Tareq in Bristol. Tareq walked everywhere to save money. Apparently, this was something students did. For me, walking? Not so much. On my visits to Bristol, I was always on a mission to cram a complete university social experience into three days and walking was a waste of valuable time.

'I came to Bristol to party, not to walk,' I complained one evening, quite loudly, and I was never allowed to forget it. *Did I mind walking from the taxi to the bar? Were stairs a waste of my valuable time?* It went on for years.

I would return from those weekends to the house in Quarrata, which was dark and quiet at night, and where the intensity of the atmosphere was the opposite of college. It was all the hard work and pressure with none of the releases of student life. No silly fun, no lifelong friendships being formed, no women, sex or romance. And you were figuring out a lot of stuff for yourself.

In my second year, I had come off the bike at speed and taken the skin off my thigh. I didn't scrub the wound properly because doing that was more painful than the injury. The wound was taking weeks to heal and got infected. One night, I finally accepted I needed to scrub it because the pain was keeping me awake. At night only the riders were in the house. The team lived in town.

I went downstairs in the darkness as quietly as possible and found what I thought was the medical supplies, took a bottle of disinfectant and sprayed it on my wound.

And duly hit the fucking roof.

I had never experienced pain like it and that is saying something. I jumped around the room in mute agony, like a mime artist on acid, trying not to wake anyone up. And then, like a genuine, MENSA-accredited genius, I sprayed some more on. The pain wouldn't subside, let alone end. I was puffing out breath to avoid screaming the place down. I took a closer look at the bottle, which looked like it was an Italian disinfectant, and realised it was household bleach.

Any university would be glad to have him.

I found myself slumped on the floor thinking that this summed it up. While my friends were making their youthful mistakes in the wrong pubs, bars and beds of university life, I was making mine here, in darkness and silence and all alone.

Bodyweight was a big thing in the Academy, because the races were so hilly. In my second year, I still wasn't finishing races. Rod said to me, 'Maybe you just need to lose a bit of weight. You're doing everything else right.'

Talking to youngsters about weight loss is a delicate matter. Rod got it just right. 'Here's what I think you need to do. Every second day, instead of your bowl of pasta for lunch swap it out for a yogurt and some fruit. Let's do that for a couple of weeks, see what happens.'

What happened was that I lost three kilos and went from not finishing a race to finishing. For Rod, that was job done.

'Good work, Alex,' he said.

Hmmm, I thought . . . *If I lose another three kilos, I'll get even better.*

But I discovered that's not how it works. I skipped breakfast, made my dinner portions smaller and my performance on the bike dipped. We'd have regular skin fold tests (where they take a pinch of fat in various places, add it all together and come up with a number) and the aim was to be between 35 and 45 millimetres. I'd got myself down from 50 to 42 and decided I wanted to get under 35, because we don't do things by halves. But if you're training hard and not eating enough, your body starts burning up muscle and turns everything you eat to fat because it's panicking. I got fatter. I learned the lesson and went back to plan A.

In Rod we trust.

Rod Ellingworth was the best thing about the Academy. In the darkest times, he was the only good thing about it. But at the end of 2008, he left and was replaced by Max Sciandri. Max had ridden professionally from 1989 to 2004, initially as an Italian, then taking British citizenship. He won Bronze for Team GB in the individual road race at the '96 Olympics.

The new training programme lacked intensity and tensions rose in the camp as we worried that we were looking down the barrel of being kicked off the Great Britain team and the end of our careers.

No matter how well or badly you were going, Rod Ellingworth focused on everyone equally. Max would focus only on the riders who were good in the moment – and going to make him look good. Under Rod, we started training at 9 a.m., with Max it was 10 or 10.30. Rod's sessions were hard and long. Max's were so easy we got bored.

What I noticed most about Max was his inability to deal with people other than the few riders he loved. Rod trained you hard, but also took the pressure off you because he put time and emotional intelligence into thinking about how to get the best out of each individual rider in his care. Sciandri didn't seem to know how to train us, but expected us to be brilliant and lost interest in anyone who wasn't.

You put trust in people, especially when you're young, to progress you as an athlete. You presume they know best and want the best for you. In my opinion, based on what I saw and experienced, Max Sciandri was not up to the job as a coach, and certainly not as a mentor.

I was in the bunch next to Erick Rowsell on a training ride one morning. When it rained in Italy, the air was warm and sticky and the skies were low, grey and fast-moving. Even the bad weather out there was painterly, which was not something you could say about Manchester. On a muddy downhill our front wheels washed out. I went down and smacked my chin on the floor. It split open. I couldn't see the damage.

'You're all right,' Erick said. 'You can ride home. But don't touch it.'

The blood was dripping onto my shorts and my front. I taped it up and was taken to the hospital. They cleaned it up, a nurse held my chin together and the doctor put three staples in. Easy.

'Come back in a week and we'll take the staples out,' he said.

A week later the skin was starting to grow over the staples and I asked Max about going back to the hospital to have them taken out.

'No, no, I'll get a friend, who is a Doctor, over to do it here.'

'Okay.'

But nothing happened over the next few days and as I examined the skin growing over the staples I got agitated. I had no car and we weren't allowed to take the road bikes into town because they had no locks and were worth so much. That evening, with no sign of Max or his friend, I tried to take the staples out with a pair of scissors. When that didn't work, I went down into the mechanics cellar and used a pair of pliers, but when I tried to pull the staples out, I realised they don't go straight in; they go in and fold up underneath, so they weren't budging. I tried to put a bit of thread behind them and pull them out, but that made me feel sick. I came to the conclusion they probably had to be cut to be taken out. I found a set of cable cutters and sized it up. I needed to nip the staple with the ends of the cable cutters and hope they didn't slip as I did it because I was putting some force into them. I lined the cutters up to the middle of the staple in the mirror, closed my eyes, and squeezed the cutters hard and that way managed to cut all three staples and then pull them out.

'We don't have to go to hospital,' I told Max the next day 'The staples fell out last night.'

I started the final Academy season well with two good results in Italy and then I steadily declined as the season went on. I got 11th in the Individual TT at the European U23 Championships, which was nothing more than okay. I was the top-placed British rider. Unlike the rising star, Marcel Kittel, who won, I was stagnating and watching my career slipping away from me before it had started.

In a bid to improve performance, rider weight was all we could focus on, and the dinner table in 2009 got absurd. We had a cooking rota and guys would cook a big bowl of pasta which no one would touch. We'd pick the chicken out and eat that, and not much of it, because everyone was worried about weight and we didn't need to worry about fuelling for training, because training was so light. The food would sit on the table in between us and we'd avoid eating it or talking about it. Morale and energy levels fell off a cliff.

We needed guidance and wisdom, an arm around the shoulder, and to eat more. Rod would have recognised what was going on and supported us. Max just sent me home.

'You're no good to me for the U23 Giro, so just go home. I'll see you at the U23 Worlds.'

That was my experience of his mentality. *You're no good to me right now, so get out of my sight.* I went home, back to Essex, back to eating normally. Back to riding the Essex lanes with Andy Lyons.

The first thing he said to me was, 'You look terrible.'

'Cheers, mate.'

We rode out across flat, exposed windswept lanes and abandoned airfields to the Blue Egg café, where hundreds of cyclists of every conceivable ability stop for the sort of fry-up that would have any team doctor reaching for his Vape. We didn't talk much. I just wanted to breathe in some home air and take in the sight of the roads and countryside that I love so much. The hour to the café from home is one of my staple rides, and Andy and I have spent thousands of hours on the bike together out there, tearing the crap out of each other on the road. That day, it was welcome mental therapy to be out there with him.

As we locked up the bikes, he took a hard look at me, pinched my stomach and rolled his eyes.

'You're eating everything on the menu.'

We took our seats inside and he let rip, appalled by my physique. 'You're stick thin and producing less power,' he said.

I opened up a bit about training and life under Sciandri. A couple of nights later, he and I went out with a group of friends, and it turned into a big night out. We ended up in a club dancing. I was trying and failing to get off with a girl I'd met. Andy was drunk like the others and leaping around. We left the club at 2 a.m. and I told him I'd drive him home. 'I've had one beer Andy, six hours ago,' I said. Which was true. We got in my car and before I drove off, I took out a whey protein drink I'd prepared before setting out for the night, because I was going training at 8 a.m. I started to drink it and realised Andy was watching me.

'Training tomorrow?' he asked.

'Yeah. Early start.'

He smiled to himself but said nothing. I drove him home. He thanked me for the lift and as he got out of the car, he looked in at me and said, 'You don't need the Academy.'

I met up with my old coach, Steve China, and went back to basics with him. For nutritional expertise, I turned to Jan Dowsett, aka Mum. Her approach was groundbreaking: three meals a day, normal food, plenty of it. Off the back of Steve's training and Mum's cooking, I went up to the National U23 Championships and won the time trial. Andy Tennant was second, Russell Hampton fifth. As so often, Andy had been right.

I also called my old sponsor at junior level, Colin Cleminson, and he put in a call to Axel Merckx to talk about me. Axel, the son of Eddy Merckx, ran Trek Livestrong in the States. Axel called me. There was no small talk or messing around; it was a very brief call.

'What have you won?'

(If you want to picture me on this call, imagine a dog panting eagerly and sitting on its hind legs.)

'The Richmond Grand Prix and the National U23 Championships,' I told him.

'I've never heard of them,' Axel said. 'We'll see how you go at the Worlds.'

And with that, he was gone.

The next day, I got a call from John Herety, who ran the UK's best domestic team at the time, Rapha Condor. 'The Academy is useless for you now,' he said. 'Your talent is not being maximised there. I'll give you a spot next year. How much money do you want?'

I had never had a conversation about money in my life. In the Academy, I was being given enough to live off, £58 a week to cover food.

I said to John, 'I don't know. I'm just looking for an opportunity here.'

'Alex, I'll give you £5,000.'

'Right. Okay,' I said, sounding like Jeff Bezos.

'Between us, you're worth £8,000.'

'Oh. All right.' I didn't know what I was doing.

The next phone call was from Max in Italy and to him I did know what to say.

'Hey, I heard you won national race,' Max said. 'Get yourself back to Italy, come do some races.'

'No, Max. I'll see you at the Worlds. I'm not coming back out to Italy. This is working for me here.'

A couple of weeks later, I went to the Worlds in Switzerland and finished seventh in a 33km TT, a race in which I grew stronger by the minute and which suggested to anyone watching that I was capable of more. The winner that day was Jack Bobridge. My finish was GB's best result ever in the U23 World TTs and the next best academy rider was Andrew Fenn in 45th place. But more significant than that, to me, was that I beat all of Axel Merckx's riders on Trek Livestrong.

A few days after I got back from Switzerland, Lois and I had a joint 18th and 21st birthday party. From the moment that Lois was born three years after me, Mum was planning this event. By the evening of the party, the Academy had offered me another year, but I felt contempt for Sciandri, whose interest in me had been revived by two great performances that had come about after he washed his hands of me.

The party was in full swing when Axel Merckx called again. Because of the time zone differences, he rang me at 10 p.m. by which time I was a teeny-weeny bit drunk.

'Yeah!' I yelled, above the music.

'Axel Merckx, have I caught you at a bad time?'

'Nah! It's a great time.'

'Okay, Alex, you've got something. We'll give you a spot on Trek Livestrong.'

What's that thing that happens in films when the person in frame stays where they are but everything arounds them moves away? A contra zoom? There's a good one in *Jaws*. And there's a cool one in that old Mafia film, *Goodfellas*. This was mine. As I stood in the middle of the party holding my hand over the phone and doing a little dance, mouthing the word *YESSSSSS!*, everything around me just fell away.

'How much money do you want?'

'Eh?'

'Money,' Axel repeated. 'How much do you want?'

I pulled myself together. Money. Right, I'm ready for this. I know what I'm doing now with money. I know my worth. I'm in control of this.

'You're the last rider through the door,' he added, 'so there's not much budget left.'

'Okay, well . . .'

I did the conversion in my head. £8,000 was roughly $12,000.

'I want 12,000 US dollars.'

The line went stony silent.

Then Axel said, 'Oh cool, yeah, I can definitely give you that.'

NOOOOO!!!!!!

I went looking for my sister. As she saw me weaving between people (because we have *that* many friends) to get to her, she smiled at me, curiously.

'Who d'you get off with?' she shouted, above the music.

'No one.'

'What's that grin for, then?'

'Got some news,' I said and led her outside.

She screamed when I told her. We hugged and jumped up and down and spilled a lot of beer. From the garden, we phoned our parents, who were upstairs, hiding.

'You sure?' Mum said. 'Or are you just drunk?'

'I'm both.'

I ran upstairs. Mum generously held back her fears of me going abroad. Dad asked questions I didn't yet have answers to. All I knew was that I was signing for Trek Livestrong. Nothing else mattered.

That was a good party. That was a tremendously good party. That night was all the parties I'd missed the previous three years.

John Herety very generously allowed me to step away from the agreement I had to join Rapha Condor because he knew Trek Livestrong would be a better opportunity for me. When I made the call to GB to say I wasn't taking up their offer for another year at the Academy, they were also superb.

'It's a great move Alex. Look, we'll still support you,' they said.

And they did. Financially, I remained on their books while I was in the States. With that and Trek Livestrong putting the team up in a house in Boulder, Colorado, I would finally have enough, more than enough, to live on. It was a new lease of life.

It took me a while to understand how much I had to thank the Academy for. It was a bear pit – intense, fraught, sometimes demoralising – but it taught me invaluable lessons about riding faster and about myself. It prepared me more than I would appreciate until I left and went somewhere else.

I had struggled in Italy, but the struggle was important. In fact, it was the whole point. It made me resilient. I wasn't good enough as a rider out there and I was too young and isolated to realise that Italy, specifically, did not suit me. I would learn, in time, that I was a far better rider than I was ever going to be in that country. I was not built to go uphill. Had I been racing in Belgium or Holland from 2007 to 2009 I would have been flying, but I would not have developed or toughened up. Those years in Manchester and Tuscany hardened me and provided me with the tools to be a professional cyclist. I didn't have a good time at the Academy but I thank it for getting me ready, and I thank Rod Ellingworth for doing it with a human touch as well as an expert one. If he hadn't had me washing cars, I would not have been headed for the States.

Since then, when I've experienced hardship, whether it's a training session or a stage race or a period of tough weeks, my ability to get through it is because

I can look to the end and know it will be worth the hard work and suffering. The Academy gave me that ability to withstand the dark stuff and the pain and get through to the other side.

These were things I would come to appreciate about those times once I got some distance. But for now, I couldn't wait to get out of there. I felt that I was being rescued from the dark, lonely castle of Quarrata.

My knight in shining armour?

Mr Lance Armstrong.

6

THE UNIVERSITY OF LIVESTRONG

Riding for a Legend, 2010

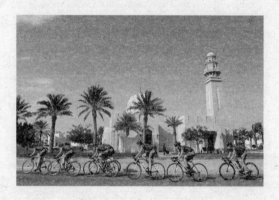

Instead of university, I went to Colorado for a further education in cycling. And my head of faculty would one day turn out to be the biggest cheat of all time. The Trek Livestrong team was created for a rider called Taylor Phinney by Lance Armstrong. The name was an amalgam of Lance's bike sponsor and his charity.

I should have been more scared to leave the UK behind and with it the haemophilia care that had underpinned my life, but the move to America was too exciting and liberation from the Academy too good for any doubts or worries to take root. Livestrong sorted out my visa and when it arrived I saw that it came under the category of 'athletes and circus performers'. (It was a mistake to share that nugget with my family and friends.)

In the fall (see what I did there?) of 2009, I flew to Tucson, Arizona for the RadioShack and Trek Livestrong meet-and-greet training camp. At the airport, I met three teammates who had flown in from New Zealand and Australia: Jesse Sergent, Ben King and Timothy Roe. Together we headed to the camp and, because of the previous three years at the Academy, I was nervous about meeting the guys with whom I was going to be training, racing and living under the same roof.

Mary Grace, the lady who organised all the logistics for the team, greeted us like she was our mum and called us 'y'all'. She was friendly and brilliant at her job. Two of my new teammates came straight over to me and introduced themselves as Chase Pinkham and Justin Williams. Handshakes, big smiles, warmth exuding from them. Why hadn't I joined in the group Facebook chat? Was everything okay with me? They were worried I hadn't joined in. 'It's great to meet you, you're an awesome cyclist, man.'

So, this is how it can be?

Truth is, I had seen an interaction between Justin and Chase on Facebook and hadn't known how to chip in. Chase was from Utah, Justin's from LA. Chase had written on Justin's wall, 'Hey man, really psyched to be racing with you.' Justin replied, 'Yes, man, we got some winning to do.' I had read that and thought, *Bloody hell, I'm so British, I don't talk about that.* I don't assume we're going to win races; we talk about it afterwards if we do. I am used to saying things like, *I think maybe we could do well today.*

I loved these guys the moment they started talking to me, but a part of me wanted to scream, 'DO YOU UNDERSTAND HOW NICE THIS IS?!'

I didn't. Because I would have sounded mad.

I just took it all in, wondered if I'd get to meet Lance, and acclimatised to being with a group of U23 riders who weren't out to slit my throat.

With Trek Livestrong I found a whole other side to cycling. It became fun again and, more importantly, I was competitive in races. America suited me. At the time, Armstrong was absolutely a hero to me, a man who had overcome disease to reach the top of the sport I loved and then dedicated a huge chunk of his life to the charity he had created. I had gone from thinking my cycling career might be over to spending my neo pro year riding in his U23 team. Life was a joy and that feeling was directly associated with being brought into Lance's empire.

On top of that, it was awesome to be riding alongside the extraordinary talent and personality that was Taylor Phinney, who had been world champion a couple of times already on the track and on the road. On the one hand Taylor was a cycling thoroughbred, with a mum who won Olympic Gold and his dad a stage winner at the Tour de France, but on the other he was the least typical cyclist I had ever met. He saw cycling and the world differently. Perhaps he could afford to, with his natural talent; we are talking about a kid who represented the United States at the Beijing Olympics when still at high school. But it wasn't entitlement or bravado with Taylor, it was philosophy. He had a stronger and more open-minded sense of his tenure on this planet than the rest of us, and had an appetite for life, racing, having fun and questioning fixed ideas, which I immediately loved to be around. Training, competing and living away from home could be a grind on many levels, but not if you were doing these things in Taylor Phinney's orbit.

All these experiences meant that I went into Christmas at home on a high, knowing that the next stop was a permanent move to Livestrong's home in Boulder, Colorado to get down to work.

And I couldn't have got the start more wrong.

Late January 2010, I flew from the UK to Colorado, moved in, stayed there for a week, got sick with altitude because I was an Essex boy suddenly living at 1,500m, and then went straight to the Tour of Qatar in February and had a terrible week. Eddie Merckx was the organiser of the Tours of Qatar and Oman, and he got Livestrong a place in both races. We really shouldn't have been there. It was for World Tour teams and a couple of Pro Conti teams, not U23s. We were so far out of our depth it was absurd. In the opening team time trial, we finished last – and then some.

I still look back on the first road stage in Qatar as one of the biggest missed opportunities of my career. It was pan flat and defined by the sort of crosswinds that decimate the peloton. Two guys attacked, Geert Steurs and Wouter Mol, and I was on their wheel. Instinctively, I got out of the saddle to go with them, but then I hesitated.

You've had a rough week, been sick, I told myself. *Sit in the bunch, look after yourself.*

Steurs and Mol were laughed at when they attacked in the headwind. They made an advantage of 22 minutes. At the finish line, they still had an advantage of two-and-a-half minutes. Then the wind dropped for the remaining five stages and they took first and second in the GC. I would have finished third, or higher, on the day and overall. It still haunts me.

But I didn't do that and we finished last as a team. When that happened Axel got an email from Lance. There was nothing in the main body of the email. Just in the subject line, which said, *Last. Seriously?*

Fuck.

That email made me shiver. I was scared of Lance and I still hadn't met him. But I guess that's exactly how he liked things to be.

That we shouldn't have been there was evident from how good the rest of the year was, competing at U23 level. Taylor Phinney won a lot and filled us with the belief we could win too. More often than not, one of us would finish second to Taylor, but we'd be there in the mix and the racing was a blast. Taylor lived in Boulder. The rest of us were a bike ride away from the university campus. We had two Ben Kings on the team, one Australian, the other American. They disliked each other, which made it even funnier. Australian Ben King, Tim Roe, Jesse Sergent and myself lived together in one part of the digs. Tim and Jesse had girlfriends. Ben and I didn't. Taylor called us 'sad' and took us to a house party and introduced us to people, and by the end of the night I had a girlfriend.

She and I took a walk together through town the following Sunday and there was a particular moment when we stopped at an intersection and I realised that from the spot I was standing on I could see cyclists, hikers and joggers passing through town, a yoga class taking place beneath the crystal-clear blue sky and men trout-fishing in the creek. The foothills of the Rocky Mountains – the Flatirons – rose into the blue to the west and the Great Plains spread east.

I'm living in a playground, I thought to myself.

There were no bad views in Boulder. There were very few rainy days. And while it's true that the winter winds could feel primordial, even they were exciting.

It was a young person's fantasy of healthy outdoor and alternative living mixed with unhealthy, full-on college partying.

It was a great year, on and off the bike, a world away from the depressing long, lonely hours in Manchester and Italy where we didn't have a social life and we merely tolerated each other. And yet, it was as I developed as a rider, in Colorado and across the US, that I appreciated what the Academy had done, what it was supposed to do – teach me how to be a professional cyclist. My Livestrong teammates had no idea about a lot of things I took for granted – like how to properly warm up for a TT, how to do an interview after a race, how to take care of myself physically and mentally. That was always Rod's intention for the Academy, to prepare you for professional cycling.

In every race Livestrong went to, we were competitive. We travelled all over the US to places I would probably never have seen otherwise, let alone raced in: New Mexico, Utah, Oregon, New York State. It was fantastic.

And it was all thanks to our inspirational leader.

There was no relationship with Lance. I saw him twice in the whole year. Once, he was doing something on stage in a town and we had to go and stand behind him. He said: 'Hello', I shook his hand, that was it. The other time was at the start in Tuscon. It's the only time in my life I've been starstruck. I had no idea what to say. Lance had these cycling shoes that looked very much like Bonts, which I wear. I looked down at his shoes and said, 'Are they Bonts?'

For a moment, Lance and I both looked at the enormous white tick on his shoes.

'No, they're Nikes,' he said. He sounded almost terrified of my stupidity.

That was the sum of my conversation with my then hero and five-time winner of the Tour de France, the man whose sponsorship with Nike was one of the biggest and most well known in the sporting world.

If I made any impression on him at all, it was as the village idiot.

Unlike my small talk, the racing got better as the year went on and that was largely down to the Taylor Phinney effect. He raised us up with him, made us believe in ourselves. I regularly came second to him, but that was like winning.

We headed to Europe for some races, starting with a stage race in Holland called Olympia's Tour, which had been won for the previous eight years by

Rabobank, who considered it their possession. We rolled up and took first, second and fourth in the TT – Taylor, Jesse Sergent and myself respectively. The Dutch media's response was that it had merely been a time trial, which is what Americans, Brits and Anzacs like, but wait until the crosswinds and sprints and then see what happens.

What happened was that we protected Taylor and he won four of the seven stages that followed. What also happened was that on one of them, Stage 4, I broke my shoulder blade.

It happened in the feed zone. Usually, feed zones are put on an incline where the pace falls off and it's safer to grab the bag. In Holland, though, it's flat everywhere, so you grab a feed bag at 55km/hr (34 mph) in the full chaos of the peloton. I'd ridden towards the soigneur and then ridden away to take the bag at arm's length. The soigneur was quite inexperienced, as was I. He panicked, then swung the bag out and dropped it into my front wheel, stopping it dead and flipping me over the top of the bars. When I went to sit up, I saw that I'd skinned my knees. *That's going to be sore*, I thought. I then tried to push myself up to standing and a sharp pain cut through my right shoulder blade.

I knew my race was run. They carted me off to a haemophilia hospital in Nijmegen. When I go away to race, the team back-up car carries my Factor VIII and a book that contains details of all the good haemophilia hospitals in the world. Nijmegen was one of them and was within a couple of hours' drive. On this day, as on so many others, I got lucky.

The X-ray revealed the break. It was 20 May and we were eight weeks out from the European Championships. This was my make-or-break year, my last as an U23, and I had to go pro at the end of it. Doing well at the Europeans was essential. The twilight world of leaving the U23s without a pro ride and having to look for one while not racing on the World Tour was one I did not want to enter.

I knew I had to be back on the bike quickly. I was in great shape, my collarbone aside, and could not afford to lose that. Mum and Dad had driven over to Holland from Essex to watch the prologue and now, within a day of getting back home, they turned around to come and get me and drive me straight from Nijmegen to the Royal London. There, I got good news. The shoulder blade didn't need surgery. I'd broken it cleanly.

Seven days later I returned to the Royal London for a check-up. The people there are always fantastic, but on this occasion I was seen by a nurse who talked to me like I was six years old. I asked her about timelines for my recovery.

'I'll be straight with you,' I said. 'I have European Time Trial Championships in seven weeks' time, and I need to be ready.'

She snorted. 'You're not even going to be training for that by then, let alone competing. You're being absurd.'

She didn't quite pat me on the head, though she might as well have done. But her condescending tone was the best thing that could have happened to me that day. Red rag to a bull.

'Absurd,' she repeated.

You don't get it, do you? I thought.

I was back on the turbo that evening, seven days after the break. On day 12, I was back on the road. The beauty of a shoulder blade break rather than the collarbone was that I could put all my weight on my hands. I couldn't stand up on the bike, but I could sit on it and pedal like hell from there.

Training with a broken bone, I turned to an old friend for a bit of security: the Maldon 10. Because I knew every metre of that route, my mind was free to monitor the pain in my shoulder as I trained. I was heading out early, the light low on the late spring Essex landscape, the fields glistening with dew, and the air cool and refreshing. It felt familiar and welcome. I worked hard, obsessive in my desire to prove the nurse wrong. The team in Colorado suddenly felt a hell of a long way away and so did the European Championships. So, I trained like a lunatic, drawing on every drop of resilience the Academy had given me, pushing myself to the brink of what my shoulder could take, tweaking my grip and position fractionally to be able to stay out longer when the bone began to argue with me.

I went back in for another check-up and was seen by Dr Dan Hart. He had taken over from Dr Colvin as my specialist the previous year and this was our first major test.

'How is it?' Dan asked.

'It's pretty good. I've got a good range of movement and it's improving each day.'

'Okay.'

He drew up a chair in front of me and looked me in the eye. 'Are you training, Alex?'

I nodded.

'Right. Hmm.' He just kept looking at me, totally neutral, no expression. Then he said, 'Are you training on the road?'

'Yes.'

'Right. Hmm. And you know, if you crash again, you could seriously ruin your shoulder? Irreparably.'

'Yes.'

'Okay.'

'It's just . . . I need this.'

He nodded. 'Okay.'

I took my Factor VIII every other day. Dan put me on to daily doses for the period the bone was knitting itself back together. And in doing so, and not grounding me, he gave me a chance to keep my fledgling career on track by making it to the most important race of my career so far.

The defining feature of the 2010 European U23 Time Trial Championships for me was that Taylor Phinney was not there (he is not European) and so the possibility – the inevitability, you could fairly say – of finishing second to Taylor Phinney was not there either.

Traditionally, the Europeans are held in classic cycling countries like Belgium, Italy and Holland. In 2010, they took place in Ankara, Turkey, which was a schlep. GB that year had a lacklustre set of Under-18 and Under-23 male and female cyclists, few of whom, they believed, could medal. So, they decided that instead of sending the normal squad of 20 they would just send me.

Me.

A one-man Team GB.

The downside? I felt slightly exposed by carrying the flag single-handedly, to add to the pressure of racing for a pro contract.

The upside? Given there was only myself to fly out there, along with one coach who was also acting as director and mechanic, the budget stretched to business class and putting us up in the Crowne Plaza, both of which were luxuries unknown. And having a huge hotel room was handy because the roads in Ankara were too dangerous to train on so I, like most of the other riders out there, did all my prep on a turbo trainer until the roads were shut off on the day before the race and we were allowed to ride the course.

The course was similar to a British TT but lumpier, the whole thing being straight out and back on a three-lane motorway. As I recce'd it with the Irish team, they complained about their hotel. There were three of them in a room so cramped they had to put their suitcases on their beds and move the beds together to make room to put a bike on the turbo trainer, which they then had to take in turns.

'Where are you staying, Alex?'

'At the Crowne Plaza. It's a fair old walk from one side of my suite to the other.'

'Bastard.'

Later that day, I was out with Dan Hunt, from Team GB, and we got collared by the chief organiser of the championships. He went for Dan.

'Hey, what does GB think they're doing? It's one of the biggest cycling nations in the world and you send one rider to our event.'

Dan was polite but firm. 'Well, if you're going to put it in the middle of nowhere, what do you expect? We had to get two flights to get here, it's two flights to get home. It's an unnecessary logistical nightmare and only you know what's motivated you to do it.'

July is the hottest month in central Turkey. I rolled out to the start line in blazing heat, 51 days after breaking my shoulder. I was on the Trek TTX with the GB Squad's Zipp wheels. I went flat out. I was never out of the big ring and never out of the tribars. I was doing 60–70km/h downhill or 40km/h uphill. When the heat got to me a bit I'd back off, then go hard again as soon as I felt I could. I did 31:08 for the 25.9km. Geoffrey Soupe of France came in 14 seconds behind me and that got him a Silver medal.

I had performed like a man possessed.

Absurd.

Winning that race was massive for me and I took my time on the podium afterwards to take it in. When I started cycling, the experts at the Royal London Hospital warned me that a bone break is one of the worse things an adult haemophiliac can have. It was always something I was scared of, but I had put it firmly away to the back of my mind so that I could get on with being a rider. To have come through this particular injury, this break – to have trained with it, got strong again and surprised a few people – was another step towards claiming my body and my life as my own, and not allowing it to be the property of the disease.

Dan Hart would have locked me in a room and thrown away the key if he had thought I would kill myself participating in this sport at this level, or if he had thought trying to train through the injury to get to Ankara was not worth the risk. He believed the dangers were acceptable when weighed against any haemophiliac's attempt – and right – to pursue their life's ambitions in the same way as people without disease can do.

I was still very young and selfish and thought about this win purely in personal terms. But the sense of pride and relief, and, frankly, of pure joy on that podium at overcoming that bone break to make it there and win was planting the seeds for a set of ideas and ambitions that would one day extend beyond myself. As my 22-year-old brain took in the thrill of victory that had seemed impossible 50 days earlier, I believe my thoughts were just beginning, faintly, to turn to all the haemophiliacs who did not have brave and forward-thinking people supporting them, like I had in Dan Hart. How could we reach them and help them?

After the event, the same official who had berated Dan Hunt for GB's one-man team, sought us both out. He grabbed Dan's arm. 'Fair enough,' he said. 'Congratulations. There's only so many Gold medals up for grabs and your team has won one of them. So, fair enough. Well done, guys.' I thought that showed real quality.

The days that followed offered me some travel time in which to sleep and reflect. The victory was taking a while to sink in. I had finished seventh in the World U23 TTs and 11th in last year's Europeans, and now I had improved to win Gold. How could I get better? What could I learn next from Livestrong and from Taylor? After two days back in the UK, I had a long flight to Oregon to further consider these things while resting up.

The Cascade Cycling Classic is possibly a race you've never heard of, but most of North America's top cyclists and teams competed in it, and it was one in a catalogue of great memories for me in my time with Livestrong. We stayed in a host house, put up by a local family. It tended to be pretty wealthy families who did this, to have a house large enough to accommodate a team of 10 staff and riders. We lived and ate with the family, went off to races and spent our downtime back with them too. I thought it was a great experience at the time. Looking back, it was a rare privilege.

Oregon is one of the most beautiful places I've visited thanks to the day job. The route along the Cascades Mountain Range took in towering pine forests and high desert. For that alone, I will remember the race, but the real reason it sticks in my mind is because of an encounter with the rider Jesse Anthony, which served to remind me that cyclists are bonkers.

I had raced Friday morning in Turkey, got unwell with heatstroke Friday night, flew home Saturday morning, had a family barbecue to celebrate the win Saturday night, drank more than is advised for someone with heatstroke, flew out on Sunday morning to the other side of America, landed Monday morning, got no sleep on the Monday because I was jet-lagged, and got no sleep on the Tuesday because a cat came and jumped on the bed and woke me up. Come the prologue on the Wednesday night, I was utterly fucked.

It was time for another key lesson in my cycling education. I had written myself off for the TT prologue because of all the above, but I went hard because that was the Livestrong way. The general team bonhomie and Taylor's inspiration meant we knew only how to race flat out. But when I got to the finish line, instead of peddling all the way through and pushing my bike out the line like I would do normally, for the only time in my career, I let off the power 10m from the line and rolled across. I finished second to my teammate, Jesse Sergent, by 0.8 of a second. I had to take it on the chin because you can't be that guy saying, *I would've won it, had I not done this.* Jesse deserved the win because he didn't make a mistake, while I did. And he went on to ride for RadioShack for many years and medalled at the Olympics and Commonwealth Games, so any win he got was always down to his talent.

But, in reality, in the privacy of my own thoughts, I was livid with myself.

You total, utter arsehole, Dowsett.

I don't know if it was tiredness that allowed me to make that mistake, but I've never repeated it.

Driving home from the race, one of the team bikes fell off the roof of the car and went under an articulated lorry behind us. Axel brought the bike back, holding it in his arms, and as he got closer I recognised that it was the bike on which I had just won the Europeans. Demolished. Trek sent their newly released model for me, which just added to the sense of a whirlwind week. The bike was great, but I wasn't used to it and with the final stage of the Cascade not being a time trial, I wasn't expecting anything from it – other than the enjoyment of riding a bike in Oregon and being on this team.

It was a 27-km rolling circuit which included a horribly tough steep switchback and a ramp of 10+% before stair-stepping to the top of the KOM (King of the Mountain) climb. Five circuits for 83 miles (144 km). It was above 30°C when we started and 38° by the end of the second lap. I was in a split of 25 riders at the front of the field.

Rod Ellingworth taught me once that in a race you have to imagine you've got one big effort – and once you've used that, that's it. You've got to be smart in road races. I used that one big effort in the Cascade to make sure that we didn't miss that break, because my teammate, American Ben King, was in the Best Young Riders Jersey and I wanted to keep him there. With that job done, for the rest of the race I just sat in the bunch thinking, *My race is done, I've done a good job, I've been useful to the team.*

With 6 miles (10km) to go and the final climb upon us, I told myself that if I could scrape over that hill intact, I'd have a look at the finish and see what happened, go with the flow, not think about winning, but see what happened. When I got over the summit, I was still with the front group, so I attacked on the downhill and got a gap with Jai Crawford, who wouldn't work with me. We got caught, but then I went again with another rider, Jesse Anthony from Kelly Benefit Strategies. He was a sprinter. Crawford had bet on the others dragging me back in so he could save himself for the sprint. But Jesse Anthony and I built a gap of 15 seconds with 1 mile (1.6km) to go.

I knew Jesse was a sprinter and I was breezing along very happy at the thought of getting second place to him. And then something happened that maybe you have to really love cycling to understand. Or am I kidding myself, and is what happened between Jesse and me indicative simply of the fact that cyclists are fundamentally, mentally, a breed apart?

He pulled up next to me and he said, 'Hey man,' with his big, thick, lovely American accent. 'Dude, I'm a sprinter so I'm going to go back to the peloton and do the bunch sprint.'

I stared at him in disbelief. We were side-to-side, turned to face each other, going at 60km/h towards the finish.

'Are you insane?' I said.

I couldn't believe what I was hearing. He was a sprinter, I am not. This race was his. But he didn't want to win a race, he wanted to win a bunch sprint, because that's his measure of success. Beating other sprinters is what makes him get out of bed in the morning.

He grinned at me. 'I'm a sprinter.'

I didn't want to talk him out of it. I said, 'Right, yes, that's a good idea. I'm not, so I'm going to see what I can do here.'

'Cool. Good luck, man. Great ride.'

He eased up and fell back into the peloton and I crossed the finish line punching the air.

After the race, Axel was in the car rolling across the finish line, assuming nothing had happened when the race announcer called out the result. He was gobsmacked. He walked up to me with this incredulous grin and asked me what had happened.

'I don't know. I won the race, but I feel like I was given it.'

A win's a win, but it didn't seem like a fair win. I told him how I had won. He roared.

'Only in cycling,' Axel said. 'Seriously, only in cycling!' He slung his arm around me and laughed again. 'You won, Alex. No one else did.'

I knew that now was the time my future had to take shape. If my race-winning form didn't earn me a professional contract now, it probably never would. RadioShack were going to take on only two riders and Taylor was a shoo-in. The chances of the other slot going to a European seemed slim. I'd heard vague noises about Team Sky showing interest in me after the Tours of Qatar and Oman and, after my win in Turkey, those noises became a rumour. But I didn't dwell on the rumours because I was enjoying myself too much at Livestrong and didn't want to cloud the limited time I had left there by being weighed down by obsessive, wall-to-wall worries about turning pro.

That said, when the offer from Sky came in, I could finally admit that it was what I desperately wanted.

It was late 2010 and Team Sky was where any ambitious young Brit wanted to go. Formed out of the euphoria and momentum of British Cycling's 14-medal haul at the 2008 Beijing Games, and with the architect of that success, Dave Brailsford, at its helm, Team Sky was not only James Murdoch's ambition for a world-class British sports team with his corporation's name on it, it was the mothership of marginal gains and the team to ride for if you dreamed of riding for Team GB at London 2012.

Joining Team Sky meant lining up with Olympic stars Bradley Wiggins and Geraint Thomas on a team that had provoked all the established teams on the World Tour by declaring its intention to win the Tour de France within five years, while operating a zero-tolerance anti-doping policy.

Who didn't want to be a part of that?

Once that contract was signed, I put it to one side and concentrated on enjoying my remaining time with Livestrong. I started doing even better in races, riding on instinct, having some fun and doing some real damage in the saddle with the team.

The atmosphere at Livestrong got better and better as everyone who was due to turn pro got a contract. Guys who were borderline got offers too; that was the Livestrong effect. I looked forward to all the races, knowing I was in a team that could be competitive in every single one.

Then we went to the Worlds and even there, with us racing in different national squads, the Livestrong riders felt the team identity. The two Ben Kings, just about the only people on Trek Livestrong who didn't get on, carried that into the championships. They wouldn't work together, they just chased each other. The coverage was hilarious, with Ben King chasing Ben King and the peloton chasing them both. Taylor came third in the road race, won the TT. Livestrong riders featured in everything and there was this weird, unspoken, brilliant feeling that even when we were riding for our countries the Livestrong victories counted more for us.

And guess what? In the middle of this fantastic flying year – with a dream move to Team Sky in the bag – returning to the GB Academy to ride in the French classic stage race the Tour de L'Avenir (unique in being a stage race raced by national teams) made being on a bike miserable again. Almost instantly, life went back to that slightly depressing stiff environment, with everyone snapping at each other and everyone out for themselves.

The Tour de L'Avenir is the U23 Tour de France. Taylor won the prologue; I was second. I saw Taylor being interviewed at the finish line.

He said, 'How did I do?'

The reporter said, 'Oh, you won it.'

'Oh good. Who was second?'

'Alex was.'

Taylor smiled. 'Ah, poor guy,' and he chuckled because it had happened so many times.

Stage 3 was 150km from Saint-Amand-Montrond to Cusset. Taylor crashed on a wet, slippery descent in the closing 15km. He was still on the floor when I passed him. I took a good look, saw that he was okay, and took no pleasure in beating him this way. But I did have the remainder of the stage to think about the fact that, having started the day second behind him in the GC, I was headed for the overall lead and wearing the yellow jersey.

It was a milestone. A really nice one. I knew it would be for only a day, because there were mountains ahead, the next stage finishing with a double climb to reach the top of the Col du Béal, but like so much of that Livestrong year, wearing the yellow jersey in the Tour de l'Avenir felt great.

With hindsight, it was almost certainly one of the early ingredients in me thinking I was destined for stardom, but it's a bit too early to broach that subject.

I was roomed with Tim Kennaugh, whose career would be cut short by a serious thyroid problem, and he was wise beyond his years. He was outspoken and saw things for what they were. From the GB Academy perspective, the entire team featured only three times in the whole Tour. Firstly, when I finished second in the prologue and wore the green jersey. Secondly, in the first road stage, when we were meant to be teeing up Andy Fenn to sprint, I looked around, found no one from GB anywhere, so I sprinted and was ninth. And thirdly, when I wore the yellow jersey. Without those three moments from me, GB didn't feature.

At the end of it, in typical Academy style, there was a squabble over how to split the prize money. Everyone voiced an opinion, mostly to split it evenly. Then Tim Kennaugh spoke up.

'You know what? Everything we've achieved in this race, Alex achieved, and none of us did a single thing to help him in any of it. In my mind, it is totally Alex's choice what happens to the prize money, but I think he should take the lot.'

Bear in mind, none of us, Tim Kennaugh included, had a pot to piss in.

I said, 'No, no, we'll split it evenly.'

What else could I say!

But I thought a lot of Tim for that. He went on to coach and his brother Peter, a Gold medallist at 2012, retired in 2019 and has since spoken beautifully and articulately about his physical and mental battles. I respect them both massively.

That taste of the Academy in the middle of my Livestrong experience cemented for me the knowledge that for me to perform at my best I needed to be happy. I don't deliver when I'm miserable. I'm not a Beat poet. I had a notion in my head which I called morale training. It was simply my understanding that I was a better athlete if I occasionally cut loose; that the monastery approach of the Academy did me no good at all.

I have always benefitted from having forward-looking, left-field thinking people close to me, chiefly my parents and Dan Hart. Now I was benefitting from Livestrong's trust in us to have freedom but not abuse it. I learned that what made me happy wasn't breaking out and partying regularly, but that once in a while enjoying a blowout was brilliant for me and my performance. I didn't need to worry about overdoing it because I had no desire to; my desire was to be at my peak. I always wanted to do what was best for me as an athlete and the occasional night out was an essential part.

Reed McCalvin was our soigneur. He lived in Boulder. He was like our dad. We didn't see much of Axel other than at races, but we saw Reed all the time. He set us all up in America. If we got into trouble, he'd be there to help us. We all had weekly massages at his house. He was an ex-military guy. He was very funny. When we first arrived in America, he said, 'Oh, we've got you all king-size beds.' We were very happy. 'Awesome, Reed, thanks man!' What he meant was there was a king-size mattress on the floor of each room and not a lot else. He took great pleasure in seeing our faces. We all loved him.

Isn't that how it should be when you're a young athlete learning your trade and trying to get in the best shape of your life? Helped by trusted grown-ups with a sense of fun as well as consummate professionalism wanting the best for you, protecting you and allowing you to have a laugh because their expert opinion is that you being happy and healthy is vital? That's what the year at Trek Livestrong was to me. We trained and raced like fury because we were happy.

The job of a soigneur can be incredibly stressful and overburdened. They do everything for the team. Reed was unflappable, even when the demands on him seemed impossible. But he had spent some years in the military and seen some things that put life in the saddle into perspective.

I asked him once, 'How come you're never stressed out by the job, Reed?'

He shrugged and smiled. 'No one's shooting at me anymore.'

It was the best year of my life. Obviously, that carries more weight if you're 82 not 22, but still, I was back in love with cycling. And it was all thanks to the cyclist who was destined to become the biggest pariah in world sport, because few things in life are ever straightforward.

7

ON PLANET DAVE

Team Sky, 2011–2012

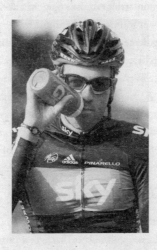

'You need to stop time trialling. You won't get anywhere just being a time trialist.'

I was given this advice by someone at British Cycling in 2006. They had sent her to my school to put me through a series of endurance tests after my participation in the scouting programme had been barred, due to British Cycling's insurance policy not covering haemophilia.

For a few agonising weeks, I had lived with the prospect of my dream being taken from me. The person putting me through my paces on judgement day was Helen Mortimer, a downhill mountain bike world champ. I did well and she told me that, given my state of fitness, there would be no problem with insurance.

'You're good to go, Alex,' she said.

The widest of smiles took over my face, and then fell off when she told me to stop time trialling.

Five years later, it was my time trialling that got me a place on Team Sky where Helen Mortimer was now working as Operations Manager. At the first meet-and-greet camp in November, I went over to her.

'Remember what you said to me?'

'Yeah,' she said. 'And what do you think?'

'That you were right,' I told her.

She was. You need more strings to your bow than the TT to have a sustained career on the World Tour. You needed them just to get within a mile of Team Sky. Helen had challenged me to be more than a time trialist. Having proved at Livestrong that I was, my reward was a place on the most exciting, challenging and, in some ways, controversial team on the World Tour.

Riding in the Tour of Qatar with Livestrong the previous year had given me a taster of the step up to the World Tour. A lot of people warned me that the jump from U23 to neo pro was a big one, and that it would take a season or two to settle in. Finishing behind the gruppetto in the Tour of Andalucía did nothing to settle my nerves, but that result proved to be the exception and straight after it I started to perform and earn my place.

On 17 April, 2011, at the Vuelta a Castilla y León, everyone at Team Sky took to the start line of the final stage wearing blood red Oakley Jawbone glasses in support of World Haemophilia Day. That was a proud moment. I was, by then, an unofficial ambassador for the World Haemophilia Society. They had an event at Silverstone which I couldn't attend, so I spoke to the Sky PR chief Fran Millar and asked if there was any chance I could wear something red on that day. The response I got was incredible. Oakley jumped on board, offering to mark the day by supplying the whole team with sunnies in a blood red custom colour that wasn't available to buy. The Sky Velo Club, which is made up of members of both the team and Sky Television, said they would do the Marmotte sportive that year in support of the Haemophilia Society, with all that money going to haemophilia charities in Bangladesh.

As I waited at the start line, I looked to my left at Chris Froome in his blood-red sunnies. Chris saw me and smiled. For a split second I saw the wheelchair that sat in the reception area of my primary school, in case I needed it.

'Nice one, Alex,' Ben Swift said to me, as he passed. By the time I'd looked round to acknowledge him, he'd gone – and so had the wheelchair.

We dominated the day. I was sent up the road in a break of nine after 80km. It was an ultimately doomed breakaway, but it put the sunglasses in the spotlight for the majority of the race and gave the commentators a talking point, which was perfect. The sheer pride of the day spurred me on and, just when the bunch expected me to fade, I dug two huge efforts out of the bag to keep me and my blood red sunnies at the front. We held a three-minute lead with 30km to go and were pulled back only in the final 2km, setting up a climax which Ben won, with a great sprint finish in Medina del Campo.

It was a great day; the best of being on Team Sky.

And yet, the team didn't bother to find out much about my haemophilia. Dr Freeman took no interest at all. I first realised this when my roommate at the Vuelta a Andalucía, Lars Petter Nordhaug, walked in as I was giving myself an infusion and nearly fainted.

'Whoa, what are you doing? Shit! No!'

Sky had said they would inform the whole team about my condition, my medication and the protocols, including the fact that I self-inject every other day. But Lars had no idea.

When it came to how much to talk to teams about my condition, I never wanted to overstate it, partly because we didn't want to scare teams off. All my career, Dan Hart and I have adopted the mantra, *I'm like anybody else until something happens.*

I thought Sky would want a bit more of a relationship with Dan and I know that Dan was amazed that Sky didn't want a meeting or a call with him to discuss everything, especially a head injury where I might not be conscious and able to tell them what to do. They didn't even ask for Dan's number.

The lack of engagement was mind-blowing, but I let it go. I suspect that all people with a rare disease experience a certain dual personality, formed by the inevitability of having to acknowledge the illness in many instances (otherwise you'd die or, at best, not make sense to people) but also recognise all the times hiding it is smarter. I missed out on so many things as a child until my treatment became preventative that when I realised Sky were not going to take ownership of my disease and treatment, I feared that explaining it would talk them out of having me on the team. So I became the Alex who never mentioned it unless it was absolutely necessary; the professional, adult version of the boy who hid his bleeds so that he didn't miss out on a holiday and didn't have to go to hospital.

In mid-May, we headed out to the Tour of California where I was an instrumental part of the leadout trains when Greg Henderson and Ben Swift won their stages. On my first year with Sky, being a part of those stage wins felt better than winning myself. I knew I was staking my claim as a team player. But having done so, adding a victory of my own for the team became my focus. I didn't keep them waiting long.

After coming fifth in the Tour of Denmark, I won Stage 5 of the Tour Poitou-Charentes. It was 171.4km and the whole team led the sprint into Poitiers. We were fast and aggressive and we split the peloton inside the final 10km with racing that opened my eyes to a whole new level of team riding. Mick Rogers and Greg Henderson towed me into the crosswind and set things up for me. I attacked 3km from the end and held on to finish 6 seconds ahead of the sprint, which my teammate, Davide Appollonio, won. Crossing the line first for the win, I felt that we had all won the race, not just me. And that felt so good. Dave Brailsford and the coaches at Sky were on another level when it came to making a team that gelled and worked like hell together on the road. There were moments of synergy between us in my first stage win as a Team Sky rider that, frankly, left me breathless.

Mum and Dad had driven out to France to watch and had taken up position near the end for the last two laps of the stage. They saw me in the mix on the penultimate lap, then next time I went by, in front.

'That was Alex!' Mum screamed.

Dad said, 'No, it can't be.'

Thanks, Dad.

We've got a great photo from the finish line of me, Mum and Dad hugging. It's a real beauty.

I became British National Time Trial Champion for the first time in my career on 4 September, 2011, and later that month came the proudest moment of my neo pro year, winning the time trial in the Tour of Britain for Team Sky while wearing the GB national champion's skin suit. Third place in the Chrono des Nations behind world champion Tony Martin was the icing on the cake of a first year beyond my and the team's expectations. I had won three pro races. I had slotted perfectly into Team Sky's leadout train. I had stepped up.

I enjoyed going to races. I can't ever remember not feeling good about work. I felt open-minded and didn't care what team went to a race because everyone was so good. There were no dull teams at Sky and no unpleasant ones. It was a multicultural team and every rider's way of approaching things was allowed to flourish. It took me a while to get used to how abrasive and forthright the Australian riders were, and how open they were beneath the gruff exterior. Greg Henderson loved the sport deeply and was great to have on a race. The older riders were happy to help wherever they could and created a positive environment. Jeremy Hunt was like a 70-year-old man in the body of a 35-year-old athlete. He was immersed in the traditional cycling world, had garnered experience from a variety of teams and knew racing better than the directors. We had to do a strength and conditioning test where they traffic-lighted you on core strength and flexibility. I scored 80%. Only two riders scored 100%, meaning they needed zero work done on them; Edvald Boasson Hagen was one of them and Jeremy Hunt the other. And that was sobering to us younger bucks who had not realised his capability.

The rules at Sky were strict, but not unusual. The fundamental one was that you were never late for anything. I can't tell you what the consequences of a rider being late were because it never happened. The division between the A, B and C teams was also stringent. After I broke my elbow and couldn't race, I asked if I could go out to Tenerife to train with a bunch of riders who were out there. It's not just that the answer was 'Absolutely no chance', it was considered a dumb question. A neo pro does not train with the A squad. The rules and boundaries did not stop it being a great experience, but there's no way Sky possessed the fun factor of Livestrong or its spirit of fearless camaraderie.

I roomed with Bradley Wiggins at the first whole team training camp and unless I spoke, we would sit in silence. Nothing. Zilch. He simply would not speak. He didn't even grunt. If he was doing something that did not require movement, like watching TV, I'd want to check for a pulse. It was a long week, but sometimes I had to stifle my laughter because I was coming from a functional, happy family where we, you know, talked to each other, took the mickey, laughed at ourselves and each other, and were kind. Soppy I know, but I recommend it wholeheartedly as an approach to other human beings. It works a treat.

Team Sky was not devoid of enjoyment, though, not by a long way. It was different to Livestrong, but good in its own way. I was often with the same riders over a series of races and there'd be the older guys and a few of us younger ones, and we got on well. Us younger riders were the C programme and the older riders were helpful and open (even Wiggins, in the right mood) and they always answered our questions and shared knowledge. The older riders would be happy for our achievements as we gradually chalked them up. There was an easy atmosphere around the meal table – the acid test for any team on the road – and I would sit there and feel secure in the knowledge that this was the best possible place to start my pro career.

I would always get a second opinion from Andy Lyons when I had a problem at Sky or was doubting myself. I would message him and other mates back home a lot, because being away on a stage race has plenty of boring moments with people who, however well you get on with them, are not your closest friends.

Andy and I are from the same part of Essex, we've ridden bikes on the same roads for years and we get each other. Sometimes you just need that familiarity and ease and trust. I was out on a ride with Andy and mentioned I was having knee problems. He looked at how my shoe plates were set for me by Sky and said it was all wrong. He had been setting his own equipment and positions for decades, having to work it all out for himself and live with the results. He changed my shoe plate set-up, gave me a small gain and solved the problem with my knees. I am fascinated by the fact, which I have experienced many times over many years as a pro, that you are employed and coached by some of the greatest minds in sport (and Dave Brailsford is, on some levels, a truly brilliant mind and a genius) with massive resources backing up their ideas and methods, but there are always things that they neither know nor understand, but which amateurs do.

In time, Andy would learn new things from the peloton via me, in nutrition and aerodynamics, but I wasn't there yet. Back then, the advice was all one-way. To be a good professional cyclist you need a mixture of the expertise of a pro tour team, and the nous and savvy of a club rider who has worked most of it out for him or herself.

'What's Brailsford like, then?' Andy asked me.

I laughed under my breath.

'What?' Andy said.

'He's not what I expected,' I said.

In those days I was, as I have mentioned, a slave to my fears of what people thought. That close season after my first year at Sky, a week or so before I met up with Andy, I had been invited to the Braveheart Cycling Fund dinner in Scotland to present an award. It was a very boozy night. I tweeted at five in the morning about being the last man standing.

The following day, Dave Brailsford texted me to say that was not the image Team Sky wanted to be putting out. 'Have fun but don't put this image across.'

It was totally reasonable of him and he was probably trying to help me, guide me, but at the time I was consumed by anxiety at the thought that I had disrespected my boss.

Those levels of fear about what people think have subsided over the years. But back then I very much cared what Dave Brailsford thought of me, wanting to ride for him for many years on Team Sky and Team GB. He was a great of the sport and I wanted him to make me one too. And the problem was that the message he sent that day, ticking me off after a night out, was as good as it got with him. The only communications from Dave were negative ones. There was never a single message or conversation when he said *Good job* or *Well done* or *Unlucky*. I plucked up the courage to ask him, face to face, why this was.

'You get the same from me as everyone else, Alex,' he said, exuding charisma. But then I was surprised when he added, 'It's something I'm working on.'

What I found tough was that, as a fairly straightforward young man raised to respect his elders, the person I most wanted to please at Team Sky was the boss. I thought my approach to hard work and my results had pleased him, but got a confusing sense that things were more complex than that with him. How hard is it to say, *I'm pleased with this* or *I want you to work on that* or – now hear me out – *Well done* ?

I maintain that my first year was the best first year any neo pro had ever had until Ethan Hayter. Not only was there no positive feedback from the boss, but when I thanked him for the three grand pay rise I received from Sky at the end of that first year, the team responded by explaining it had been given to me in an administrative error, but that I might as well keep it. Now, years later, that makes me laugh (albeit that squirmy, uncomfortable laugh you get watching Ricky Gervais in *The Office*), but at the time I felt stupid and belittled for thinking that a good season would end with a smile and a pat on the back.

Still, all that crap was taking place off the bike, not on it, so I was very excited about my second year with Sky, not least because of the arrival of Mark Cavendish. Quite apart from the experience and raw ability he would add, I was psyched by the prospect of being part of his leadout train. Riding for Cav at Team HTC–Columbia had made better cyclists of Mark Renshaw, Matt Goss and a man I looked up to massively, Tony Martin. I wanted a bit of that Cav effect.

But my 2012 season got derailed very early, in March, in Belgium. Sitting eighth in the GC on the Three Days of West Flanders, I broke my elbow. Michael Rogers and I had done well in the prologue and on Stage 2 we were entering a wet cobbled section when a rider in front of me crashed and took me down. The rider was Leif Hoste and I already had my own views about him, which were shared by much of the peloton. Those opinions were confirmed two years later when the Belgian cycling federation brought a doping case against him and he got a two-year ban. Already convinced he was a cheat, I felt a disproportionate anger towards him as I lay on those very hard cobbles.

You've wiped me out and you shouldn't even still be in this sport.

My elbow hurt badly. The team got me back to the bus and tried to assess the damage. I was scared that I had done something serious and made the decision to get myself home. I had driven to the race from the UK, because it's easier to drive to Belgium from Essex than fly. Driving back was not the right thing to do, but I was scared about having surgery in Belgium and got in a panic about getting back to Dan Hart at the Royal London. That was my safety net. That was my second home.

I was also young and unwise and more concerned about my car than I should have been. Team Sky were sponsored by Jaguar at the time and I had this absurd £90,000 Jaguar XKR, which scared the shit out of both me and my dad because it handled like a dog. But you make hay while the sun shines and this was just the first in a very long series of bad car choices.

After I got showered and dressed, Kurt Arvesen, who had recently retired and become a specialist coach at Sky, took me aside. 'Are you okay, Alex?'

'Yes, I'm fine. I'm fine.'

'You don't look okay.'

'No, no, I'm okay.'

'Then why are you holding your arm?'

'Look, I can move it, it's fine. I'm just going to go home.'

I thought I'd just bruised it heavily. The car was an automatic and I held on to my shirt as a makeshift sling. I had to stop for petrol and get Dad some chocolate for his birthday the next day. Filling up with petrol was difficult. I had pain shooting through my arm, so I rang my old school friend Tareq, who was studying to be a doctor.

'Mate, I've hurt my elbow. Do you think it's broken?'

'I don't know, Alex. I'm in Bristol and I'm studying medicine, not clairvoyance.'

Thinks he's funny, Tareq.

'Can you move it?' he asked.

'Yes, I can.'

'Hopefully not, then,' he said.

What I didn't tell him was that when I said I could move it, I meant I could move it with the other hand. I couldn't actually move it. I had heard what I wanted to hear, absolutely, categorically, confirmed by a doctor: no break.

'Great. Thanks, mate.'

I rang my sister. 'Hey, I've hurt my elbow. It's definitely not broken because Tareq said it's not, but I can't really do anything for myself at the moment. Can you meet me at mine and help me unload the car when I get back?'

Lois was biblically hung over. 'Yes, absolutely, I'll be there. You total prat.'

When I got home, she and I got a taxi to Chelmsford hospital straight away because I was now in agony and white as a sheet. I was X-rayed and the surgeon took a look and laughed, 'Oh, yes, you broke that good and proper.'

Back home, I called Dan Hart. 'I've broken my elbow and they want to operate tomorrow.'

'You're coming straight to the Royal London in the morning,' he said. 'We're doing it, no one else. Have some medication now, to get your levels up.'

'Right, okay, but my right arm is in a plaster cast from my hand to my shoulder, so I can't inject myself.'

'Alex,' Dan said, 'someone has to. You need to do it now. Your levels need to be high before we cut you open. Do you understand me?'

'Got it,' I said and hung up.

I looked at Lois who was lying on the sofa, shipwrecked by her hangover.

'Went out last night, did we?'

'Popped out for a bit, yeah.'

'Good time?'

'Not really. I got dumped, so I went out to drown my sorrows.'

'Lois! Why didn't you say?'

'I think you're in a worse state than me.'

'Well, funnily enough, I think we're about to find that out. Just had an interesting chat with Dr Hart,' I said to her.

She looked blankly at me, through her unkempt hair. 'Huh?'

'Dan says I need medication now,' I said and waited for her to cotton on.

She was barely able to focus. I watched the cogs turning in her mind. But, no, nothing.

'You're going to have to do this.'

She leapt up off the sofa. 'SHIT! WHAT? NO!'

Lois had never had to inject me. Why would she have had to learn? My mum did it. Doctors did it. From just before my 10th birthday, I did it. Seemed like there would never be a scenario in which she'd needed to do it. Why would there be? Well, now we had the answer: it would happen when I had one arm in plaster and my parents were having a romantic night away.

This might be the right time to mention an anomaly about my dad. He has never and could never and will never inject me. He is so scared that, frankly, I wouldn't want him to try. I'd rather ask a passing stranger. When I was a kid, Mum and Dad were trained how to inject me intravenously. It was going to be something that I would need doing a lot. Mum was fine straight away. Dad was skilled in theory – when the nurse made him inject a piece of fruit – but could not put a needle in his own son. It wasn't that he felt a bit squeamish or didn't fancy it or couldn't be bothered. He wanted to be able to, wanted to play his part like he did in everything else to do with my care, but he was physically unable to puncture my skin with the needle. He's my hero. He has done everything for me, been there every inch of the way, but he has never injected me because he physically, mentally cannot do it.

'You're going to have to inject me, Lois.'

My sister held up her shaking hand and presented it to me. 'No, Alex.'

There's a Mark Twain quotation I like: *Get a bicycle. You will not regret it if you live.*

The only other time I was seriously worried about my haemophilia was half a decade later at the Tour of Poland when I crashed badly, took a chainring to my neck and found myself looking down and watching my navy blue Movistar top turn burgundy. I knew I was in trouble and bleeding pretty hard out of somewhere.

A paramedic came over, looked at me a little bit wide-eyed. 'Are you okay?'

'You tell me,' I said.

Then I started panicking, because I couldn't see where the bleed was and he didn't seem to be able to tell me. The only thing more scary than a bleed is a bleed you can't trace.

The wounds on my neck were a series of neatly spaced horizontal and vertical lines. The problem was that the crash had happened 300m from the finish of Stage 1 at the height of a bunch sprint, when your heart rate is really high, up in the 180s, when blood would gush out of even a paper cut.

The chainring slashed my neck open close to some pretty important arteries. I was very lucky it didn't go any further. I tweeted a picture of my injuries with the words *Quiz time: Campag, Shimano or SRAM spacing anyone?*

These moments were bound to happen; that was the unspoken acceptance when an athlete and a doctor agree to go forward with that athlete's competitive career. I had arrived in Dan Hart's clinic in 2009 as someone with an unusual trajectory for a severe haemophiliac. All he knew, when he took over my care from Dr Colvin, was that I was an accomplished young cyclist. He had never had a patient who was participating in sport at that level. What he immediately understood about me was that there was a competitive gene in me, and a love for wheels and speed. And he understood not only me but us as a family from the start. He got that I was driven.

My first substantial conversation with Dan was a phone call on the eve of my departure to join Trek Livestrong. He was a cycling fan, used to watch Phil Liggett commentating on the Tour de France, and he was personally interested in having a cyclist on his list.

'Do you understand how extraordinary you are?' he said.

Dan considered me to be on the cusp of something remarkable. He envisaged it bringing pressure into my life and getting attention.

'My job is to keep your expectations of achievement moving forward without haemophilia obstructing them. That has two sides to it: you being allowed to do everything you are aiming for and avoiding medical complications that would derail your career. That's my role.'

Dan firmly believed that for many years my physical strength had protected me as significantly as the Factor VIII medication. And we both agreed that if you are cycling at 60mph (96km/h) down an Alpine pass, the risk to your health is not from haemophilia but from coming off.

It is not safe to crash if you don't have haemophilia.

Dan felt pressure in those early days of my career. He had self-doubt. *Am I doing the right thing? How many of my peers would encourage Alex and support him even though he is putting himself at risk?* This was the beginning of the era of personalised care for haemophiliacs rather than a one-size-fits-all approach. I am very lucky indeed to have received it. There was new flexibility in how to approach the treatment of individuals. Dan advised that my prophylactic treatment would have to reflect the intensity of my training and racing and the amount of risk, so that instead of just taking my preventative medication every other day, there would also be extra Factor VIII when training was intense. On race days, I would always have it. It was this decision that would mean I didn't bleed to death in Poland.

And to be clear, Factor VIII is not performance-enhancing. In no way, shape or form or under any circumstances or in any volume does Factor VIII enhance or aid performance. It is a chemical that anyone who is not a haemophiliac produces naturally and which stops you bleeding uncontrollably. I don't have it, my liver does not produce it the way yours does, and synthetic Factor VIII gives me what everyone else has. I need more of it on days when the chance of a high speed or high volume crash is higher because those are the days when the risk of a bigger bleed is higher.

Taking Factor VIII does not make me faster or make it easier to go faster. And it won't enhance your performance either.

Got it?

The dosing I take gets me near to a non-haemophiliac's natural levels of Factor VIII, especially in the first four hours after infusion. It means that, effectively and for a short while, I don't have haemophilia. A good illustration of the way my medication works is this: if I take Factor VIII on a race day morning and no further dose the next day, then by the time I am in a bunch sprint on that second day I have severe haemophilia again – and in a high-risk situation, that means I'm totally unprotected.

The protocol, set up by Dan early on for race days and high-risk stages, has hardly changed in more than a decade. Dan is without ego and sees his job as being to facilitate and make safe as possible my fully committed pro-cycling life. Dan keeping things steady with an *if it ain't broke, don't fix it* approach, using standard medication that has been around for years, has been great for me. There's been a load of new medicines coming on the scene and I'm lucky: Dan doesn't want to be a clinical rock star grabbing headlines for himself.

But he does want to get what we've achieved together noticed, as do I, purely so that we may advocate for other sufferers to live more fully, to participate in sport to whatever level they choose, having the same opportunities as non-haemophiliacs.

Together we faced challenges getting my charity, Little Bleeders, through the Charity Commission with the old fold who believed that cycling was not a good sport to promote for haemophiliacs. We've lobbied government to get equal support for haemophiliacs across the country. We want fairness and equality for sufferers everywhere in the UK, and beyond. It's illegal for a doctor to cut off haemophilia medicine to a child if they want to play football, but that's precisely what happens in some parts of the UK. We help those people, advise them of their rights, and direct them to doctors and hospitals who understand haemophilia care better, those who know that it has been lifted out of the Victorian era by preventative medicine.

Livio di Mascio has been my upper limb orthopaedic surgeon at the Royal London for many years. He has always taken the same attitude as Dan to my treatment. Whenever I have landed on his operating table, he has recognised the importance of getting me back on the bike. Livio's view is that haemophiliacs are capable and need to push on, not hide or stagnate. I count my blessings to have an insightful and forward-thinking NHS surgeon. Dan Hart calls him a legend – and rightly so.

Because I was *first in family*, I was always going to be detected and diagnosed later on, when the evidence that something was wrong reached a crisis point. Game-changing advances in the last decade mean that preventative treatment is now given in the first months of life to known haemophiliacs and immediately on detection for *first in family* haemophiliacs like me. The arthritic damage to my elbows and ankles is like pouring paint stripper on your car bonnet and hoping you'll get the sheen back – if the paint stripper is blood and the sheen is the joint surface. One big bleed is enough to take the sheen off your cartilage and that predetermines premature arthritis.

My broken elbow in Belgium was a paint-stripper moment and I have arthritis there now and cannot straighten that arm. It was also indicative of another trait of haemophiliacs – their extraordinarily high threshold for pain. I am in no way unusual in that respect, nor is it something that applies only to sport. Most haemophiliacs can bear high degrees of pain because pain was their first and formative life experience.

Thanks to Dan Hart, and Brian Colvin before him, my elbow break in Flanders did not leave me bleeding to death. It was painful and would ruin my second season at Sky, but the only problem it left me with was the simple task of persuading my baby sister to jab a needle into my vein.

She was standing opposite me, showing me her trembling hands and refusing. I got the medication out and gently coaxed her to sit down with me.

'I'm not saying you have to do it, but let's talk it through.'

'But what if I kill you?'

'You can have my bikes.'

'Really?'

'No. Just imagine you're putting the needle into an orange but put it into that spot right there. That's the vein.'

I thought it might take 10 minutes to talk her round. Her hands were still trembling but – and this is my sister to a T – she just let out a kind of pissed-off sigh, rolled her eyes and did it, put the needle in perfectly. First time. Straight into the vein. Then blew her fringe out of her eyes and smiled.

We didn't tell Mum and Dad about my injury because they were away for the night to celebrate Dad's birthday. But once I was at the Royal London next day I filled them in and then went into surgery. Fixing the elbow went fine. I was sent home after five days of observation. A week later, I was on the turbo trainer, but I was useless. I felt shit. My elbow started swelling up badly, then my hand swelled up too. I was rushed back into hospital and as I lay there beginning to think that my dream of London 2012 might be in danger, Mum, Dad and Dan Hart were discussing the possibility that I could lose my arm.

I had a *Staphylococcus* infection and they couldn't immobilise the infection that was on the metal plate inside my elbow. Without the plate, antibiotics and a blood infusion would have cleared the infection, but because there's no blood supply to a metal plate we had a bigger problem. The only sure way to clear the infection was by removing the plate, but the bone was still broken so that was impossible. The only route to take was six weeks of antibiotics until the bone had healed enough to remove the plate.

I was in hospital for the first two weeks. The antibiotics were done intravenously and they were burning the inside of the vein, so they kept having to move the port around, four times a day. There were 16 tablets a day of antibiotics when they let me go home. I was off the bike for two months and had four operations in total. It was a bad time, a very long and drawn-out injury that made a massive dent in the season. And it destroyed any hope I had of going to the Olympics in London that year.

8

TREADING MY OWN PATH

Team Sky to Movistar, 2011–2013

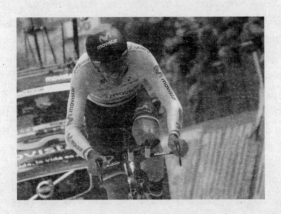

In October 2011, at the end of my first season, Rod Ellingworth and Sean Yates had called me in and said that I would do a Grand Tour in 2012. It would likely be the Giro.

'That's exactly what I wanted to be told,' I said. 'Thank you so much.'

I was delighted. It was the natural progression.

Go forward to the spring of 2012. Soon after I started training again following the Flanders injury and *Staphylococcus* infection, I knew my place was in doubt. But when I asked Sean about the prospect of me going to the Giro, he said, 'You never were going.'

Not so much a jaw-dropping moment as one when you feel a shiver. 'Oh, okay, that's odd,' I stuttered. 'But, last year, when you said –'

'No, you were never in mind for the Giro.'

By the time of the Vuelta a España came around, I was fully fit and racing again.

'We're going there to win with Froome,' Sean said. 'You lack experience, so taking you would be a risk. We can't take you.'

I began to question my future with Sky. *If they're not taking me to the big races because I lack experience, then they're never going to take me to the big races.*

Chris Froome came fourth at the Vuelta. The team came fifth. It was an average showing in an otherwise imperious year. The 2012 line-up was fantastic: Wiggins, Cavendish and Froome, the extraordinary Edvald Boasson Hagen, Luke Rowe coming in from the Academy. The Belarusian Kanstantsin Siutsou, who was always instrumental in any Wiggins win, was part of a posse of talented riders, including Richie Porte, Michael Rogers and Christian Knees, aimed and trained to propel Wiggins to a first Tour de France victory. And they did.

Not only did Sky's announcement that they intended to win the Tour within five years – a statement of intent derided by many competitors when it was made in 2010 – come to fruition three years ahead of schedule, but their first yellow jersey would prove to be the start of an insane dominance of the Tour that decade. The team won 47 races in total in the 2012 season. Wiggins was incredible, not just in winning the Tour and at London 2012, but throughout the year. Cavendish won 15 races, including three at the Giro and three at the Tour. It was fantastic. But personally, something had changed.

Suddenly I felt sidelined, just like the invalid kid ordered to sit out playtime. But I wasn't an invalid, I was fully recovered and very fit indeed and had been delivering and improving for two seasons on two continents.

I got a strong sense that missing out on the Olympic Games had left me diminished in the eyes of Dave Brailsford and the Team Sky gods – even though with Wiggins and Froome taking Gold and Bronze in the TT, no one could sensibly argue that, even fully fit, I should or would have been there.

Missing London 2012 should not have meant anything to Dave Brailsford. My recovery from a big injury and my excellent form should have meant a lot. And while I was hearing: 'Meh' from Team Sky, two people called on the same day to say that the Spanish outfit Movistar wanted to sign me. One was Brian

Smith, a former British Road Race champ and commentator. The other was my manager at the time, Paul De Geyter, who had taken me on when I was at Livestrong and handled my move to Team Sky (and made no money out of me, because his policy was not to take a cut of neo pro salaries).

Movistar had history and momentum. They had been around for decades since their inception as Team Reynolds in 1980. As Banesto, they had been home to five-time Tour de France winner Miguel Induráin in the first half of the 1990s. And they were having a very good 2012, re-establishing themselves as GC contenders.

They had brought Alejandro Valverde back into the fold after a two-year ban handed to him because, without ever testing positive himself, his DNA had been matched to a blood bag in the Madrid clinic of Eufemiano Fuentes, a doctor involved in a doping scandal. They had just signed one of the most exciting young cyclists in the world, the Colombian Nairo Quintana. They had won the Vuelta a Andalucía and secured stage wins in all three Grand Tours. Twenty-nine wins in total that season would take them to fifth in the world rankings.

From the first time they made contact with me, Movistar said, 'You will go straight to the Giro.' They were very clear. They had a plan for me; they wanted to develop me.

'We think you can be a very, very good bike rider, Alex.'

Then Jonathan Vaughters at Garmin approached Paul as well and I felt there was more interest in me from outside my own team than from within. Feeling wanted means a lot to me in my professional life.

Although he didn't issue any praise himself, Dave Brailsford's sports directors had been consistently telling me that they and the boss were delighted with my performances and my progress. But now, in their eyes, the sheen seemed to have gone from me, like some of my joints. Brailsford started blanking me completely and ignoring any emails I sent him about plans and contract renewal. Suddenly, I didn't exist. That's a feeling that does not sit well with me. It feels like a very close cousin of psychological bullying. And it wasn't just me, he blanked everyone on my team.

I was sitting in my flat one evening, giving everything that was unfolding some thought. I can sometimes disappear down wormholes when I do that. One of them was my resentment at having been shipwrecked in Belgium by a fucking drug cheat. It's pathetic, I know, but if one of the multitudes of clean cyclists, virtually everyone else on the peloton, had taken me out on those cobbles, I wouldn't even have been thinking back to it. Another thought that I stewed on that evening was the memory of what Sean Yates had said to me at the previous year's Tour of Britain. Sky had gone there to win it. Geraint crashed and the team achieved nothing until the last day when I won the time trial.

Sean said at the time, 'This is our second biggest race of the year behind the Tour de France and you have saved it for us by winning this time trial.'

How could these guys not offer me a contract?

Then Paul called me.

'Movistar are getting twitchy about waiting on an answer from me. What do you want to do?'

There were risks in going to Movistar. It was an unknown for a rider like me to go to a Spanish-speaking team. And for a young British rider to leave Team Sky was unprecedented.

Movistar wanted me and had big plans for me and what mattered to me was that those plans included riding in the Giro in 2013. The offer was a good one. I felt wanted and valued by them. Pro cycling is a cattle market and being wanted by people who had a plan for me was the feeling I was after.

I sent another email to Brailsford and this time I copied a lot of people in, including my coach, Paul Manning; my new agent, Sky Andrew; my dad; and Rod Ellingworth.

> *Hi Dave, I guess from your lack of communication that you don't wish to keep me. I'll be signing a contract in principle with Movistar this afternoon. Kind regards, Alex.*

I'd like to sit here and tell you that Brailsford picked up the phone to me, but he didn't. He got his right-hand man, Carsten Jeppesen, to call Sky Andrew immediately.

'We want Alex and we'll offer him a contract today, but he's not a very good climber, so the offer will reflect that.'

Their offer was a big hike, matching Movistar's. They clearly did want to keep me. But they hadn't been arsed to reply to our emails for weeks, they had eventually made the offer in terms designed to put me in my place, and the all-powerful man at the top was showing how big and tough he was by still blanking me. Suddenly, incredibly, being at Team Sky wasn't even tempting.

Carsten had said coldly to my new agent, 'He's not a very good climber.'

Let me address that comment, because it's not accurate.

I'm a shit climber.

I'm a time trialist and a leadout man and a team player and a stage winner. I am not a very good climber in the same way that Usain Bolt is not a particularly useful marathon runner and Erling Haaland is not a tremendously gifted goalkeeper (although he probably is, the freak).

If Sky had offered me more money than Movistar at that point but in the same manner, I would still have turned them down.

I spoke to my parents as I always would. Mum was nervous about me joining a team not based in the UK where my haemophilia specialist and care was. Dad believed in going where you are wanted. I agreed with him. Mum became adamant I should stay at Team Sky; that you don't leave a powerful team. We agreed to disagree, but she wasn't happy.

I do not claim to have been better or more significant in 2012 than I was. But if your team are not remotely excited about having you and are disdainful about keeping you, how can you develop that relationship? It was not a situation of my choosing and if Sky had come in early to re-sign me and wanted to talk to me in a normal way, there is no way I would have thought about leaving that team in that era. But the extremely unhealthy dynamic of the situation was absolutely clear to me.

Sky Andrew told Carsten we'd think about it. But we didn't. Brailsford had spoken by not speaking. He made the decision easy for us. We had no doubts. Let's go to Movistar.

Dad and Mum would sometimes say, 'We'll tread our own path.' It was their way of navigating me through early life in a way that kept me safe but, at the same time, made me active, not missing out. In the era I was born into, missing out was what you did if you had what I have.

We'll find something, son.

We'll tread our own path.

Going to race in America was another such pathway. Not many people did that.

Sometimes doing your own thing has served me well; other times, not so much.

If you are excluded as a child, the fundamental concept of being alone, of going your own way, is established, as is the knowledge that people are talking about you, have an opinion about you – a truly horrible thing to be aware of as a kid. I found it far easier to learn how to inject myself intravenously than to stop caring what people said about me. Inevitably, opinions are sometimes based on ignorance. *He's the boy who could give my child AIDS.* It's incorrect and ludicrous.

Being a British rider and choosing to leave Team Sky was also something that was not done. But I did it. I did it to get more chances to ride in the major races with a Spanish team whose pedigree lay in the great European Tours. It was a new chapter in my career and at the precise moment it started Dave Brailsford announced that Team Sky would be reinforcing their zero-tolerance policy regarding doping and that Sky's coach Bobby Julich and directeur sportif Steven de Jongh had left following confessions of drug use during their racing careers.

All Movistar needed to do to create the worse possible speculation about me was to bungle the PR handling of my move. And all Movistar did do was bungle it. They announced my departure from Team Sky to join them 24 hours after de Jongh had left Sky with an open letter confessional, which was 48 hours after Julich's doping admission. Given that I have to self-administer intravenous drugs regularly on the team bus and that Movistar had seen nothing wrong in readmitting Alejandro Valverde to the team after his delayed two-year ban for his part in the Operación Puerto blood doping scandal, I desperately needed Movistar to get the timing right. Instead, they were, in their own utterly consistent way, oblivious to the outside world and launched me into the maelstrom of Sky's doping confessions.

News24 reported my move like this:

British time trial champion Alex Dowsett has become the third member of Team Sky to leave in a week, by joining Spanish team Movistar. Dowsett finished eighth in the time trial at the world championships last month, and narrowly missed out on being a part of Britain's Olympic cycling team . . . His move follows the departures of sporting director Steven De Jongh, and race coach Bobby Julich, who both admitted they had taken performance-enhancing drugs, in fallout from the Lance Armstrong scandal.

Gee, thanks. And also, FOR FUCK'S SAKE!

The *Guardian* did me more favours:

After Dave Brailsford's announcement 13 days ago that Team Sky would be reinforcing their zero-tolerance policy regarding doping, any departure from the team leads to speculation as to the reason why, particularly after the exit of their race coach Bobby Julich and directeur sportif Steven de Jongh following confessions of drug use during their racing careers, and that of their lead directeur sportif Sean Yates for family and health reasons. But if the announcement on Tuesday that the double British time trial champion Alex Dowsett is leaving to join the Spanish squad Movistar raised eyebrows, and caused brief speculation in the Twittersphere, that appeared to be down to inept PR. It seems the clumsiness was on the part of the Spanish team, who are probably not aware of the situation at their British counterparts and announced their signing of the Briton the day after de Jongh's departure from Sky had been confirmed with a lengthy open letter confessing to doping.

There was a flip side to all this, which was the speed at which the speculation died down (almost instant) and the lack of any serious rumour or questioning. What it proved to me was that no one really thought I was anything to do with Sky's doping problem. But I could have done without it. I was already feeling the pressure of having chosen to leave what was seen as the dream team for any British rider and tread my own path.

When I dared look on Twitter again, I mentioned that I needed to brush up on my non-existent Spanish and got messaged by a Spanish teacher saying, 'I live just down the road from you. If you want Spanish lessons let me know.'

Great, I thought. *That was easy. When do we start?*

I turned up and the door to the house was opened by a Spanish woman who was frosty, to put it mildly, not the helpful, bubbly woman who'd messaged me. It quickly became apparent that she was, indeed, not the bubbly woman who'd messaged me. She was the mother of the bubbly woman who'd messaged me, who was in fact a bubbly 14-year-old girl, called Natalia. Her mum was Spanish and her dad was English and he was excited about having me there. He had lined up his three daughters, the other two being older, in a neat line and introduced themselves at their father's prompting. They gave their name and their age, the older two stating plainly that they were not too much younger than me. Dad looked on expectantly.

I got very embarrassed very quickly and muttered something about 'just being here to learn Spanish.'

The dad turned out to be very funny and once he'd let go of the idea of marrying one of his elder daughters off to a Movistar cyclist, it turned out he was a cycling nut. Natalia was a good teacher and I kept going back for two years. It helped a fair bit, but there was always an issue with the fact that she was teaching me school Spanish so I could say things like *I am wearing blue trousers*, when what I really needed was to be able to talk fluently about gear ratios and tyre pressure.

I learned quickly with Movistar that the way they operated was very loose but kind of charming, like their PR. Antonio Flecha asked me how I was finding life at Movistar. He had been a teammate at Sky who barely acknowledged my existence until I proved myself in the Tour Qatar, after which we became good friends. He was just one of those professionals whose respect had to be earned, and I had no problem with that.

'Organised chaos,' I said to him.

He laughed. When Antonio laughs, it swamps his face. He exudes a certain love of life. He was the first ever Argentine-born man to win a Tour de France stage and you might remember him as the rider who mimed releasing an arrow from a bow as he crossed the line, a tribute to the family name: *Flecha* means 'arrow' in Spanish.

'That is the perfect description of how Movistar operates,' he said.

Having come from the extremely forward-thinking Team Sky, Movistar seemed stuck in their ways. My first impressions were, *How do these guys win races when this is such a charming shitshow?* Then I learned. I had my eyes opened to the fact that there's more than one way to approach things.

In those days, Tirreno–Adriatico (known rather beautifully as the Race of the Two Seas) always began with a team time trial and ended with an individual time trial. We went there in March with a strong team and it was total disarray. For the team time trial we did three laps of the course as a recon, but were told to do it at 90% race pace.

I was in the saddle thinking, *I'm taking from my race here.*

But that was how Movistar did it: they went hard and didn't organise a team order, didn't sort out length of turns or any of the other tactics you would usually predetermine for a team time trial. At Sky and Livestrong, you knew exactly who you were going to be sitting behind and what length turns you would be aiming to do.

Movistar's approach was, 'Okay, go recce the course in any order.'

Wow! I thought. *This is something else.*

When we finished the recon they said, 'Now warm up.'

Warm up? I was toasted.

Then Eusebio Unzué, Movistar's team manager, was on the bus with us all trying to decide what overshoes we should use. It was chaos, but somehow we rolled towards the start and everyone was kitted out properly and we resembled a team.

One of the riders said down the radio, 'Which order should we go in?'

There was silence.

Then, Eusebio's voice: 'Okay, this is the order. As we're in Italy, Giovanni (Visconti) is Italian, so he's going to start.'

123

That was the reasoning. Right up there with rock paper scissors.

We finished second and we beat Sky. I was in shock. We'd only lost to Quick-Step. Cav won it for them and they had been at the location for a week to prepare for the team time trial. I was already thinking, *With the way Movistar operate, would a week here have been a benefit?*

Maybe there's something in just rocking up and knocking it out.

What I also learned that day was that at Movistar there were no egos in the team. That came out in the way everyone rode. What cripples a team time trial is when someone gets on the front and they're feeling good and really kick the pace or when someone stays on the front for too long and can't hold the pace. The Movistar riders seemed to have an instinctive feel for the length of time they should do at the front, and we never dropped the speed and we never had any spikes. It was shambolic in one way, yet these guys knew what they're doing.

9

LETTING GO OF THE BIKE

The Giro, 2013

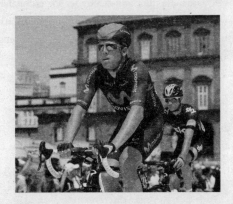

There is no such place as *good enough* for an elite athlete. There is no such thing. Our life is always about the next level. The appetite to push for more, the compunction to, is an ingredient in what sets us apart.

When we achieve something, it immediately loses its lustre. We want more. What shines is the success we have not yet achieved. We want to beat our opponents and vanquish yesterday's version of ourselves. That's why we push our bodies and minds into places of suffering and mental anguish that not every person wants to experience.

———

In 2013, I was 25 years old and had ridden for the greatest neo pro team in world cycling and the biggest name in British Cycling I was a two-time National

Champion and Commonwealth Games Silver medallist. But I had not been selected for a Grand Tour.

The three Grand Tours stand apart as the greatest, most profound tests of every rider in the peloton. The Giro d'Italia, the Tour de France and the Vuelta a España are each one of them 21 days of the most intense bike racing possible, over every type of landscape, from flat to almost vertical. The cumulative effect, day by day, on the body and mind make the Bushtucker Trials look like a Michelin-starred meal preceded by a holistic massage.

The Grand Tours are more than bike races, they are national events that have become global phenomena and cultural institutions. They are where every road racer wants to be while, simultaneously, knowing they are going to hate every day of it.

The 2013 Giro d'Italia was my first Grand Tour. To say I was excited is a sizeable understatement. To admit that I was shitting myself would only be honest.

'Are you insane?'

I had heard that a lot the previous year. Along with, 'No one chooses to leave Sky, Alex.'

Or, in some cases, 'No one leaves Sky, you idiot.'

Fair to say, it was not the case that everyone around me supported my decision to sign for Movistar. I had left the most sought-after, talked about, commercially backed and aggressive team on the World Tour. I had done it to ride in Grand Tours and the moment I was selected for the 2013 Giro I knew that decision was about to be judged publicly. It was a whole new type of pressure.

No one chooses to leave Team Sky? Maybe, but no bike racer chooses to train for a decade and watch a normal childhood and adulthood pass them by so that they can then watch their teammates ride in the big races.

The Giro d'Italia has its own unique flavour and romance. Think of it as Italian opera disguised as a sporting event. It is the least modernised of the Grand Tours, the one that still feels like an epic, chaotic race, not a polished brand. A huge part of this is down to the tifosi, the Italian crowds who line the route in even the most obscure, mountainous areas, and support the Italian riders passionately, unequivocally, sometimes demonically.

The field was exceptionally strong. My bosses at Movistar considered it the strongest in the race's 100-year history. Despite this, it was seen as a head-to-head battle between the cool, controlled, meticulously prepared Bradley Wiggins at Team Sky and the charismatic, carefree Vincenzo Nibali, riding for Astana.

Wiggins was coming to Italy as Tour de France champion and with a Giro win his stated priority for 2013.

And Nibali? He was Italian. Everybody wanted him to win.

We started on the colourful, high-walled, narrow streets of Naples, in warm sunshine, with the breathtaking sight of Mount Vesuvius to the east leaving me in no doubt as to the pure honour of being here, and the thrill. After a late, high-speed crash, Mark Cavendish won the sprint and took the famous pink jersey, the maglia rosa.

We were all up early the next morning to cross to the island of Ischia. It was a Sunday and the sound of church bells filled the blue sky as we made the crossing. I began to understand that this Grand Tour took place within the grain and culture of everyday life in Italy. There would be people making their way to church now and lining the race route later.

Stage 2 was a 17.4km team time trial – technical, full of bends and perfect territory for the superlatively drilled Team Sky to rack up points. Movistar came in second, 9 seconds behind Sky, a strong team effort and a satisfying one for me. It meant that I wore the white young rider's jersey because the leading young rider, Sky's Salvatore Puccio, had the pink jersey. Paul Smith had designed the Giro jerseys that year and he was there that evening, buzzing at having two Brits wearing his designs, myself and Cav in the red sprinter's jersey. In one of those pinch-me moments Paul gave me his number and told me to stay in touch.

On Stages 3 to 7 I got involved in attacking for some breakaways early on but did not feature significantly. I quickly understood that a Grand Tour is different to anything else and that all your previous racing was not a classroom to prepare you. Your education in competing in the Grand Tours begins when you ride in one for the first time. I was pushing myself, observing everything that was going on and loving every minute of being a part of it.

I was gaining experience of the job which Sky wouldn't give me because I didn't have enough experience.

The Giro is more complex and intimate than the Tour de France. It is unpredictable, draining and yet a continuous, chaotic shindig. The towns you pass through, and the Italians in them who somehow combine fanaticism and carnival simultaneously, take you a world away from the corporate sterility that pervades a huge chunk of the UCI World Tour and ASO's running of the Tour de France. From a bike rider's perspective, the Tour de France feels dogmatic, like a thoroughly engaging but overproduced and ultimately predictable Hollywood film. The Giro is the best indie film you've ever watched: beautiful, passionate, with breakout performances, not perfectly lit or executed but moving you, leaving you changed, stirred, in love again.

Stage 3 took us through the beautiful, intense, hairpin bends and wooded groves of the Amalfi Coast. The next day, entering Calabria, we had the first warnings of the unpredictable weather and the first of many crashes in slippery conditions. Stage 5 was almost wiped out by a series of crashes but, in avoiding them all, Team Katusha's Luca Paolini retained the pink jersey. Cavendish won his second stage the next day and, on the podium, dedicated his victory to Wouter Weylandt, who had been killed two years ago to the day, at the Giro. That was Mark exemplified – a winner and a good man.

Stage 7, San Salvo to Pescara, was seriously wet. Bikes and riders were sliding all over the place. I rolled in the bunch with Wiggins, the pre-race favourite on a self-declared mission to win his first maglia rosa, nine months after winning the Tour de France and Olympic Gold. He was in the second part of his invincible phase. In the first, he had been invincible. In this, the second, he believed he was invincible. He had been genuinely astounding in 2012, and the general mood of opinion in the peloton now was that both he and Team Sky believed this status had automatically carried over into this next year.

As we rode side by side, waiting for the attacks of the day to start, we talked about the time trial from Gabicce Mare to Saltara coming up the next day. Team Sky had been out to recon everything prior to the tour. He had ridden the whole TT and was telling me a bit about it. It was long, 55km, and that was perfect for him.

'It's going to mean there's massive gaps,' he said.

He turned and looked at me, unflinching, neither hostile nor friendly.

'Huge,' he said.

I got the feeling that he meant he was going to knock the time trial out of the park and that the massive gap he was referring to was going to be between him and me. And I believed him. Why wouldn't I?

You're Bradley Wiggins, reigning Tour de France and Olympic time trial champion. The most brilliant bike rider on planet earth right now. Of course, you're going to knock it out of the park. Of course, you're going to eviscerate me.

That clear warning aside, I enjoyed listening to him share some knowledge with me about the course. I appreciated it too. *This is cool*, I thought.

I had zero expectations for the time trial on Stage 8, which is strange when you consider that I was the national champion at the time, so had the jersey with the stripes. But I felt small compared to Wiggins and generally in awe of my first Grand Tour field of riders.

And there was another factor. What I was sitting on.

'Alex, you're giving away 30 seconds to Wiggins with just your handlebar set-up alone.'

That's what Rod Ellingworth, who was now performance manager at Team Sky, said to me at the Giro. He wasn't playing mind games; he was talking about the very different ways in which my current team and my previous one worked with their sponsors.

Movistar and Sky had more or less the same sponsors from 2011 to 2013. Even though Sky was sponsored by Adidas, the kit was made in the same factory as Movistar's, who were sponsored by a company called Nalini. I had experience of both and the quality of Movistar's kit was not a patch on Sky's.

Both teams were sponsored by Pinarello as well. Movistar and Pinarello were not one without the other. Both were synonymous with Miguel Induráin, the last cyclist to win the Tour de France on a steel-framed bicycle. He rode a Pinarello in each of his five Tour de France wins for Reynolds, the team that became Movistar.

Team Sky had joined forces with Pinarello two years earlier and helped develop Pinarello's new time trial bike, which only they could use. Suddenly our TT bike was inferior to Sky's and that was the end of Movistar's long relationship with Pinarello. Team Sky made their own handlebars, at about £12,000 a set

– unthinkable money at Movistar at the time. We had ugly, bolted-on Vision bars that weren't adjustable and with cabling that was an aerodynamics monstrosity. Wiggins' bike was clean without a cable in sight. All this, according to Rod, gave him at least 30 seconds over me before we started.

On the morning of 11 May, Movistar hadn't left time to recon the whole 55km TT. Of course they hadn't. The first 25km was technical, so we looked at the first 15km of that. There were a lot of corners and it was in fact so technical that I couldn't begin to remember it all. It was going to be impossible for the team car to tell me what I did or did not need to break for. I had to take this upon myself. So, I did what I've done hundreds of times in Britain and learned on the Maldon 10: study the route, get technical myself, make a plan, and don't make the classic time trialists' mistake of obsessing about how much power I am producing on my computer and, instead, think only of speed.

It's just you and the course. Screw the rest. Screw Wiggins. Screw Sky. Just ride your bike fucking fast and don't use your brakes.

There were a lot of corners. I didn't want to be braking for them. So, I had to know the route. Even if we had recce'd the whole route, it was too much to remember anyway. I needed a map. Movistar's sponsor, SRM, supplied us with computers that didn't have maps. The solution was obvious, I would do as Sky did and use a different computer, even if it pissed off my team and their sponsor.

I had a Garmin in my bag. I spent an hour or so plotting the route into it and then went to the mechanics.

'Can you put this Garmin on my bike next to the SRM?'

'Have you checked it with the boss?'

'Absolutely not.'

'What!'

One of Movistar's weaknesses was how beholden to sponsors they were. If a company wanted to sponsor Team Sky but didn't produce the best equipment, Sky would tell them that either they would not be sponsoring the team or, yes, they could sponsor the team but until they made something good enough Sky would use other equipment. Movistar's stance was: they're the sponsors, so we use whatever they make.

'Listen to me,' I told the mechanic. 'If you get asked, you tell them to come to me. It's on me, my decision. Just get the Garmin on my bike, please. Okay?'

'Okay.'

I covered up the Garmin logos with tape, worried about pissing off SRM – well, not worried exactly, just trying to avoid it. If I had been that worried, I guess I wouldn't have been strapping a rival piece of kit on to the front of my bike next to theirs. With every logo covered up, the thing was still bright blue and impossible to miss.

Now, having mined into the mentality that thousands of windswept, rain-soaked hours riding the Maldon 10 route in Essex had handed me, I was ready to race my first Grand Tour time trial.

The reason I had taken the ballsiest risk of my life in turning down the offer of a contract renewal from Dave Brailsford and Team Sky was to be here in a Grand Tour and up against a god like Wiggins. The only way to go at this course was to embrace the absolute love of speed that got me into this sport in the first place and to adopt an overall *don't care, not listening, la la la* ears blocked policy to the dangers of taking every single corner at top speed.

This is the Giro, for Christ's sake! Crashing is worth it.

Once I got racing, I knew pretty quickly that I could not have attacked that course so fast mapless without killing myself. There were so many blind corners with hedgerows where you have to tip the bike in and it was impossible to see if you were entering a 180° hairpin or just a kink. I put blind faith in my map and gave myself wholly to the love of speed that a bunch of a few hundred psychos in Lycra need to have in order to enter the elite ranks of bicycle riding. I embraced the *que sera, sera* attitude towards crashing that the previously mentioned group of idiots (for I am one of them) all possess and managed to pull a minute on Wiggins in that first 25km. Wiggins punctured and that cost him 15–20 seconds and the other 40 seconds I gained by riding like a man possessed.

For the first 25km I didn't know the splits, but I knew that I was overtaking people and feeling great. In the team car behind was Eusebio. It was the first time I'd had the boss following me in the time trial. It was a lot of pressure, but I was, despite all the wormholes my mind likes to go down, essentially still a cocky youngster and I didn't overthink it. I was so focused on my own performance, I wasn't thinking about anyone else's – and that's exactly where you want to be, mentally, for a time trial.

Taylor Phinney, highest paid neo pro in history, second in the World TT Championships to Tony Martin the year before, the man I was destined to always come second to, had started three minutes in front of me. At the first intermediate check, the team came down the radio and told me, in Spanish, 'The time to Taylor Phinney is one minute and 30 seconds.'

My Spanish might have been allowing me to order pizza and tell the population of Spain that my trousers were blue, but I was nowhere near being able to accurately translate a garbled radio message received at 60km/h on a bike. Not accurately at least.

I translated it as, 'You're one minute and 30 seconds down on Taylor Phinney. You're in second.'

Holy shit! I thought, *someone has set fire to Taylor's arse.*

If he's made one minute and 30 on me, and I thought I was flying, then I don't think Wiggins is going to beat him. I don't think anyone's going to beat him. Mind-blowing!

The second 26km were flat, straight roads; good territory for me. I hoofed it along and saw a BMC car ahead. Initially, I thought it had to be Adam Blythe, who had started 13 minutes in front of me. *If I've caught him*, I thought, *he's going to be in trouble for the time cut.* I knew he was crap at TT, but this was spectacularly bad. But it wasn't Adam. As I got closer, I saw that it was Taylor.

That's when it clicked in my brain; one minute and 30 seconds behind Taylor, as in having started three minutes later, not as in a further one 30 behind.

I'm ahead. Come on, Alex! Destroy yourself for this!

I passed Taylor at around the 40km mark and as I did so, he gave me words of encouragement.

Then 15km to go. There was still a horrible climb left to navigate. Mum, Dad and Lois had positioned themselves halfway up it. When David López, a Team Sky rider who looks nothing like me and is nearly a decade older than me, went past, Mum was convinced it was me and screamed at him, 'Go on, Alex!' and got a bemused glance from back from the Spaniard.

Mum already had some form when it came to mistaken identity and cheering on the wrong guy at races. She would claim, later that evening, that López was the spit of me, but evidence does not support her. On the one hand, skinny blokes in Lycra onesies wearing pointy helmets do all look pretty similar, so you want to cut her some slack. On the other, she gave birth to me, so I had always hoped she'd know my face.

I went at that 3km climb as hard as I could. The splits would reveal that I went into it with a big lead on everyone and lost a chunk of it there, but not all of it.

I went over the line fastest so far: 1:16:27 for 54.8km.

That's cool, I thought, *but there's a lot of people still to come.*

I sat in a hot seat and Movistar were brilliant at taking the pressure off. They always believed in you. They were far more optimistic than I am in a situation like that and in general. I think I'm more of a realist. Members of the team were coming up to me and saying things like, 'You can win this, we knew today could be your day' and 'No problem if you don't win this, you've already done great.'

It was a long agonising wait. There were still the likes of Luke Durbridge, the Australian national champion, and Jesse Sergent, my teammate at Livestrong who had won Bronze on the track at London 2012, to come – and they could beat me on the day. And there was Wiggins.

Wiggins went off fast and on a mission. He came through the first intermediate time check at 26km 52 seconds slower than me, having suffered his puncture. Then was the technical bit, and the long straight bits, where I expected him to pull it back but he didn't. At the bottom of the climb, I had 55 seconds on him still. Then he really rocketed up the climb. He pulled back a 45-second deficit, but it wasn't enough and I got him for 10 seconds.

Wiggins had been the last specialist to ride. At that point I realised, *Holy shit, I could win this.*

Nibali gave me a fright; he went through the first checkpoint faster than me and I knew he was a much better climber than I am. Someone on the team messaged me:

Eusebio says, don't worry about Nibali. He'll fall apart on the long straight.

That's exactly what happened.

There was no one left. It took me a few moments to take that fact in, even as my team erupted with joy around me. I had won.

I felt strangely calm. I was used to winning TTs. The gravity of what made this one different, the fact that I had won on my first Grand Tour, on the Giro d'Italia, was difficult to take in. I had dreamed of it so often since turning pro that it still felt unreal. And, in a strange way, the gravity of it never did quite register.

It's tempting as I look back to put this reaction down to me being super-humble, but I have to be honest with you. While I was immensely grateful, proud, excited and – I very much hope – my usual polite self, I feel obliged to come clean about what I was really thinking: that this would be the first of many.

I thought that if you are going to be a superstar, winning your first Grand Tour stage is simply something that has to happen. I'd had a habit of winning since I first got on a bike and this was the next level. *I'll probably win a load more and I'm really looking forward to it.*

I was still by the hot seat and grinning like a Cheshire cat when Wiggins walked past. Just before he entered the tent, he slowed down. I watched him hesitate, stop and look over at me. Then he glared at me, wiping the smile off my face but doing nothing to dampen the joy in my heart. He held his stare a moment longer, then moved on.

I'm a pretty straightforward person and Wiggins was a mystery to me. On Stage 14 of his victorious Tour de France the year before, when a spectator threw carpet tacks onto the road causing Cadel Evans to puncture and lose two minutes, he and the other Team Sky riders signalled to the whole peloton to slow down to allow Evans and the other affected cyclists to catch up. There's that Bradley Wiggins and there's the Bradley Wiggins who glares. I have no idea which one is the real him or the one he most enjoys being. We all have our demons.

One thing I was certain about, after getting the evil eye from Bradley, was that if I'd stayed at Sky I wouldn't have even been at this Giro, let alone winning at it. And there was something very Giro-esque about my mum and my sister hijacking the podium ceremony by jumping up on to it and smothering me with hugs and kisses before the traditional peck on each cheek from two Italian models.

I love a tradition, me.

I wiped the lipstick from my cheeks and sent a message to Dan Hart.

'Thank you for this, Dan.'

Dan replied, informing me that my win had only been the second biggest cycling event of the day, because his son had learnt to ride a bike a few hours earlier.

'First time I let go of the bike and Teddy cycled away without support!' his message said, before going on to offer me generous and heartfelt congratulations.

I messaged him back, agreeing that letting go of his son's bike was the bigger moment. I sent congratulations to his son and to a proud dad. I had no idea at the time that there was more to this exchange than I understood or could have imagined.

I got cleaned up and did an interview. As it finished, Wiggins came up to me, shook my hand, said, 'Well done' and left.

Go figure.

Then Taylor breezed into the Media Zone and, because he is Taylor Phinney, wrapped me exuberantly in his arms. He hugged me and, with a big, broad generous grin, made it clear how happy for me he was that I had beaten him. He did it in front of the podium and the media. It was really nice, a very cool moment he gave me.

My Movistar bosses were overjoyed. This was the best side to being on that team, the family feel of it, the love of cycling that courses through them. When Eusebio is happy, he really looks it. He has an unforgettable smile; it engulfs his face.

Geraint Thomas messaged me: 'Fucks sake Dowsett, I've done 112 grand tour stages and not won one and you've done it in eight.' Classic, sarcastic, dry Geraint, but it meant a huge amount to me that he took the trouble.

But here's the thing: all those messages from other riders and coaches helped me think I was better than I was – not that I needed a lot of help to think that.

That Giro win was one of the best moments in my professional life, but also one of the worst things that happened to my career because that was the moment I told myself, *Yes, I am up at the top level.*

In reality, I was not there at all.

I was now a member of a group of riders that could win races, but there was another group, with Wiggins, Fabian Cancellara, Tony Martin and Rohan Dennis the standout members, who were the Unbeatables, and I was not one of them. I belonged to a bunch of 20 guys who could all beat each other on our day and who could sneak a win every so often if we had a belter of a day and the Unbeatables were absent or having an off-day. That was the reality.

But that's not how I saw it.

Despite my areas of self-doubt and my general good manners that implied a certain modesty, I came to Movistar with an arrogant belief that, having been educated at the GB Academy, Livestrong and Team Sky, I knew it all. That attitude mixed with a Giro stage victory was going to prove a potent cocktail.

Mum, Dad and Lois walked back down the mountain to the hotel, carrying all the bouquets of flowers and garlands I had been given. Lois had dressed up smartly and gone quite big on the hairstyle and make-up in case there were any rich, good-looking Italian blokes around. This might also have been what prompted her presence in the hot seat area. Mum and Dad teased her mercilessly as she struggled down the steep gradient in her heels.

They went back to the hotel to start celebrating. They were staying at the team hotel. When they had booked their trip and realised their hotel was the Movistar hotel, they asked me to check with the team management if it was okay, just in case a rider's family shouldn't be mixing with the team. Movistar barely understood the question – their reaction was that of course my family should be in our hotel. They were delighted. They really were genuinely family-minded as an organisation.

Mum gave the owners of the hotel all the flowers and by the time we arrived back the hotel staff were decorating the reception with them. I wasn't sure of the protocol. We wanted to celebrate, but we had 170km and a couple of big climbs to do on the bike next day on our way to Florence. The team cracked open a bottle of champagne and I said a few words of thanks, then caught up with my sister and my parents. Dad told me that Taylor Phinney had come up to them at the start of the day and said, 'Your boy could do it today.'

Dad had replied, 'I doubt it.'

I sent Mr Bevan a message. He'd already know the result, no question, but I messaged him because he was a part of this. He was a part of the reason I had got here. I needed to thank him, but how do you begin to thank a teacher who has done so much for you?

Then the team doctor, the late and very lovely Jesus Hoyos, RIP, took me to one side.

'Alex, this is massive.'

'Thank you.'

'Do you want to go home?'

'Excuse me?'

'Do you want to go home?'

'I don't think so. I mean, what do you mean? There are 13 stages to go.'

'Well, you've won a stage. If you want to go home it's no problem at all, because our Giro's done. You don't need to win anything else, so if you want to go home, you can go home.'

I was speechless, given that I was having the time of my life. 'I think I'll stay and keep riding.'

'Okay, cool, great.' And with that, he wandered off.

I am convinced this wouldn't happen in any other team. It was the mañana culture writ large. What wasn't unique to Movistar was the way that, as with a lot of pro cycling teams, the team doctors end up running the show even though that is obviously not their job description. Not everyone managing a pro cycling team is the sharpest tool in the box, but you have to be pretty smart to become a doctor. They're naturally intelligent and their intelligence naturally infiltrates management and often they end up calling far more shots than they are employed to do.

Jesus' question to me was the ultimate *take the rest of the day off* moment and was vintage Movistar. That conversation would not have happened at Team Sky.

At Sky, if you weren't 10 minutes early, you were late. The very first team meeting I had at Movistar, I turned up at 7.23 p.m. for a 7.30 p.m. start. There was no sign of anything happening. The second in command, Alfonso Galilea, laughed when he ambled in.

'It's 7.30, what am I missing here?' I said.

'You'll learn,' Alfonso said.

The meeting started at 7.55. That is how the whole thing operated. Obviously, they all turned up to races on time, but everything that didn't need to happen on time didn't happen on time.

If something went wrong in Team Sky, there'd be a constructive discussion. In Movistar, there'd be an argument. You'd get back to the bus and find two teammates having it out with each other and then it would all be fine. No hard feelings. No egos. No lingering resentment.

I had a good evening after my win, celebrating with my team and with Mum, Dad and Lois, strictly water for me after one glass of champagne. And I bumped into Dave Brailsford in the hotel that evening. He congratulated me, just, but then he couldn't stop going on about how quickly Wiggins went up the final climb.

'Yes, I know,' I said, politely. 'He pulled a lot of time back on me on the climb. It was very impressive.'

Wiggins had done 460 watts. I hadn't done anything close to that and hadn't needed to, but I stood there listening to Dave Brailsford, watched the effort it took for him to get the words *Well done* out of his mouth and then bang on and on about how strong Bradley Wiggins had been on one climb.

And I was thinking, *What are you on about, Dave? Wiggins has just become the first man in history to win the Tour de France and the Olympics in the same year, he doesn't need bigging up. There is no sentient being on Planet Earth who thinks I am in any way stronger or better than Bradley Wiggins, but given your position of superiority in the sport and over me as an individual, to the point that you froze me out as if I didn't exist, why are you so unable to acknowledge that today was one of those rare days when we beat you?*

But that's Dave Brailsford for you, and that's probably one of the many reasons why he's been such a huge success. It's not simply that many of the greats are arseholes, but the point is that they're happy to be arseholes and don't care who sees and hears them being arseholes, because they're winners and they couldn't care less.

Wiggins pulled out of the race after Stage 12, crushed by the conditions in one of the worse Giro's for weather in its history. It is just another ingredient in the Giro's mix and adds to the drama: the race takes place in the spring and is susceptible to the bad weather that the high mountains produce. We had blue skies, hot days, the sort of light rain that creates a slippery film on the road surface, the torrential rain that causes multiple crashes, and snow.

It seems to me that most of Italy is hilly and of the areas that are not most of them are mountainous. After my stage win, the race was dominated by the high mountains of northern Italy and the Dolomites – steep, tight climbs that didn't even have the decency to be constant but dipped and rose and double-backed on themselves, adding mental torture to the physical.

But while this terrain was tough for me, I was too busy enjoying a sensational team experience and performance to care. There was also the personal joy of seeing my mate and honorary Essex boy Mark Cavendish take further wins on Stages 12, 13 and 21. As a team, we set up sparkling stage wins for Giovanni Visconti on Stage 15, in heavy snow on the Col du Galibier, for Beñat Intxausti the following day, and for Giovanni again on Stage 17. Movistar came third overall.

Vincenzo Nibali climbed through snow and a wall of baying, ecstatic fans to claim victory overall, and that was kind of perfect too – an Italian winner of the maglia rosa. The magnificent fans had got what they deserved and desired.

When I got home from the Giro in late May, and with 10 days before heading to France for La Route du Sud (nowadays called Route d'Occitanie) and the Nationals after that, I headed to the Royal London for a check-up. It was a routine appointment with Dan Hart and the first time we had seen each other since my first Grand Tour stage win.

One thing I should make clear is that, if they're lucky, a haemophiliac and their specialist do not often get to be in the same room as each other. Check-ups for me are, thankfully, few and far between, so if I stay out of trouble, our communication is mostly by phone. That's why it was a bit special that I was seeing him so soon after the Giro.

The appointment went its usual way; blood tests, a check-up and ultrasound from the physio, then in to see Dan the consummate professional, serious and efficient, finding out everything about me and from me that he needed. But there was also a celebratory atmosphere to it all, born of our journey together having taken us to that Giro win. As we finished up, I thanked him for his text message after the win and joked about his son learning to ride his bike being the main event of that day.

Dan went to reply, but suddenly he couldn't speak and turned away. For a moment I thought he'd swallowed something or was choking. He couldn't get his words out. Then I realised he was desperately trying to hold back tears for some reason.

I didn't understand what was happening.

He sat down, still trying to suppress his tears. 'Give me a minute,' he said, faintly, barely able to talk. It took him a few more moments to gather himself and then he talked – and this is a faithful account of what he said to me.

'It may seem weird how emotional this is for me, but having a young son without haemophilia always reminds me how hard it must have been for your parents to have let go of your bike for the first time and let you cycle without stabilisers, with all the concern that your Mum particularly carries with her all the time. I make the comparison in my head quite frequently when I'm doing the kids' clinic here. It's a big moment in any parent's life, taking their hand off the saddle and letting go of that bike, seeing their child cycle off for the first time or run into the playground or start at school, but an order of magnitude more profound for a family living with haemophilia. Your stage win for me stood for everything we try to do to in the clinic to help parents be confident enough to let their child go and play.'

Then he said, 'Bloody hell, it must've been hard for your parents! Amazing that they ever did that, let alone allowed you, encouraged you to race bikes. It's a bravery I cannot comprehend as a father myself, thinking how hard it must've been but never really knowing, as I haven't had to go through it.'

When Dan let go of his son's bike, at the same time that I was racing through Italy, he didn't picture his most high-profile patient riding in a Grand Tour; he thought of the same moment he had just experienced, of letting his child go on his own, and of all the haemophiliacs for whom letting go is not a next happy step in your child's progression, but a moment full of fear.

His tears were also a recognition that, for as long as I ride competitively, my parents will carry that fear of me coming off my bike around with them, just as a young parent of a child learning to ride a bike does.

My initial thought, as I sat across from this man in whose expert and brave hands I place my care, had been to presume that his tears, though unexpected, were simply tears of pride in what we had achieved together. But they were something different and more profound; a raw expression of sadness for what a diagnosis of haemophilia does to the innocent joy of becoming new parents. They were for the abject fear, the heart-in-mouth knowledge that they have to let go of the bicycle and the absolute certainty that this will mean falls and bleeds and trips to hospital and needles searching painfully for veins; that it will mean tears and pain.

He wept for the parents who have to hurt their child to make them better.

When I left my appointment, I walked out on to the Whitechapel Road and broke down.

10

THE ARMSTRONG COMMENT

The Start Line, Beijing, 2012

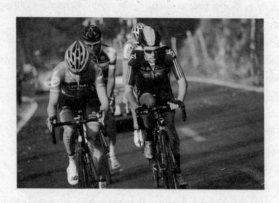

In 2012, as detailed and compelling revelations about Lance Armstrong came out, I described him as *a legend* to a reporter. It wasn't one of my finest moments. What a journalist then did with my comment perhaps wasn't one of his.

It's time to talk about needles and it's time to talk about China.

The Tour of Beijing comes at the very close of the World Tour season and, in 2012, it was my final race for Team Sky before moving to Movistar. There was an end-of-term feel for us all in Beijing, but that was ripped apart by the publication of a US Anti-Doping Agency (USADA) report that revealed Lance Armstrong to be a serial drug cheat and bully.

There were a lot of sports journalists in China for the Tour and there was one in particular who the peloton had noticed, because he seemed to be new to cycling. Prior to Stage 3, he was sticking his microphone in the faces of a lot of riders in search of a soundbite.

I was the fool who gave him one.

He went up to my teammate, Edvald Boasson Hagen, and said to him, 'Why are you in this strange T-shirt?'

Bemused, Edvald, said, 'Because I'm Norwegian National Champ.'

The journalist said, 'Wow, impressive,' and moved on.

Everyone thought this guy was odd. I saw him approach Steve Cummings and get little out of him. When he came up to me, I treated him with the same respect that I do anyone else.

'What do you think of the Armstrong situation, then?' he asked me.

I was in race mode. I hadn't read the report and its hundreds of pages; obviously I hadn't. You couldn't access any social media in China in 2012. All we'd heard was that Armstrong had been done for drugs. Without the details, this wasn't earth-shattering news, given that he was the last among the greats from his era who had not been done for drugs. While admiring his achievements on and off the bike, and being constantly told that he was the most drug-tested athlete on the planet and had never tested positive, we also felt that it was a bit too good to be true that this clean guy had beaten all of those other guys who were drugged up to the eyeballs.

I abhor drug cheats, but shared the view of most of the riders who were busy preparing to race and not reading the USADA report, that if Armstrong was being revealed as a doper, then it would be in line with, and to a similar extent to, his peers (the dreaded level playing field). We were a new, clean generation of riders and we were busy doing things differently. We didn't know the extent of the bullying, the bribery – the full works of just how bad this thing actually was.

That's why, when the reporter asked me what I thought of Lance Armstrong's situation, I stupidly, among other things, called him *a legend*.

If I had wanted to be a smart-arse about it, I could have argued in the days that followed that *legend* can be taken in more than one way; the Kray Twins were legends. But that would be dishonest because it wasn't the way I meant it. I didn't know the full story and I was referring to the heroic side of the Armstrong story, the cumulative ingredients of a level playing field back then, his achievements on the bike, his cancer, his books, his charity. As riders for

Livestrong, we had all worn those yellow wristbands and it was ingrained in me in my youth that he was a legend of the sport.

I had visited cancer patients in hospitals that were being funded by Livestrong and had seen how grateful they were to us just for being bike racers representing the charity. Lance was this huge figure, and I felt a connection with him because he had come back from cancer and I had overcome a rare disease. Those things go deep in a young man's mind and don't immediately dissolve when you are told that this man might be something else entirely.

It takes a long time to deconstruct your heroes.

That's why I said what I said. I was 24 years old and I said something stupid.

After the race, I had a few messages from people along the lines of, 'You're headline news on BBC Sport.'

Oh, that's cool, I thought.

Tareq messaged me: 'You're trending on Twitter @TheArmstrongComment.' Then he called me.

'What's happened? There's no way you said that.'

All hell broke loose. It was the first time I had ever had anything negative written about me. Journalists had always been fair with me, generous even. I was absolutely mortified that I'd done this to myself and inconsolable that I had done this to my team. It was one of the worse moments of my career.

I was fortunate that I couldn't access social media and that all I was exposed to was my friends messaging me not to do so. I was crippled by anxiety about what people thought of me and, even though I was set to leave, I felt physically sick fearing I might have brought Team Sky's name into disrepute, overwhelmed by worry at what Dave Brailsford would be thinking. I sent him a long, gushy apology and he didn't reply to it, which just added to my concern.

Steve Cummings came looking for me to check I was okay.

'I got away with it,' he said.

'What do you mean?'

'That reporter asked me about Armstrong and I was like, "Screw Armstrong. I want to talk about the Tibet situation, seeing as we're in China." But he wasn't interested.'

When I did get myself in front of some internet and news, it was bad. The BBC Newsround website reported, 'British cyclist Alex Dowsett says Lance Armstrong remains "a legend of the sport" despite the doping accusations against the American.'

A few hours later, the BBC Sport website wrote, 'Alex Dowsett, who rode for the US-based Trek-Livestrong squad, called Armstrong a "legend" for his battle back from cancer.'

Simultaneously, the full extent of the USADA report was becoming clear to me. I issued a message via Twitter and Facebook to clarify my views:

'I just wanted to set the record straight as some things have not been clear in my comments reported in the press today. When I was quoted saying Lance Armstrong is a legend, this was in regard to the charity work he has done. Also, when I said it doesn't matter, what I mean is that we are racing clean now and it is a different sport to what it was back then. I'm sorry for the misunderstanding, I was just about to start Stage 3 of the Tour of Beijing and I wasn't clear in my thoughts. I do think what Lance has done is completely unacceptable.'

I did further interviews afterwards saying I wouldn't shake hands with Armstrong, and things like that. A few people made jokes about the fact that I did a full 360° turnaround in 24 hours. I reminded them we hadn't had access to the full information.

BBC Sport updated their coverage of the comment to include my statement and apology, and my clear position on Armstrong. No one continued pressing me because no one who knew me and no journalist believed there was any more to the story than the fairly simple one that had unfolded:

I made a stupid comment about a story I didn't know the full extent of.

I was castigated for it.

I was given, and took, the opportunity to explain myself and state clearly for the record what I really believe, and in doing so I didn't try to defend the stupidity of what I'd said and I did not defend, in any way, Lance Armstrong.

That was that.

My victory on Stage 8 at the 2013 Giro came seven months after the Armstrong comment in Beijing. It was long in the past. And yet, when reporting on my first ever stage win in a Grand Tour, the *Sunday Times* journalist David Walsh chose to write this:

'The greatest surprise was Dowsett's victory. Before yesterday, the 24-year-old was most famous for his defence of Lance Armstrong in a BBC interview after the American's banishment from cycling and life ban from sport. "I don't think it matters," he said of Armstrong's doping ban, "he's still a legend of the sport." He would later change his view, admitting that what Armstrong did was unacceptable.'

I had clarified my comments within hours of making them, having participated in a 162km stage of a world tour race in between, and all this had taken place 213 days prior to my Giro victory, but that didn't seem to matter to David.

David Walsh is the sports journalist who, along with Paul Kimmage, was instrumental in bringing Armstrong down. Armstrong hated them both – and that alone probably tells you how good they were at their job.

People like Armstrong don't waste their energy on hating people who aren't a threat. The peloton regards him as a man who flips between being the self-described *fan with a typewriter* and being the sport's self-appointed FBI. He deserves huge respect for what he has done for cycling in not only exposing its worst ever cheat but doing the job so comprehensively that Armstrong has been wiped from the record books and disgraced. He placed himself in harm's way and was harassed and threatened in his devotion to rid cycling of Armstrong on behalf of us all.

He is smart and experienced. He knows what he's doing. He knows what he is writing.

Perhaps I'm less smart than him. In fact, yeah, let's just all agree now that I am less smart than him. But I do know about needles. David Walsh could have asked me a bit about that. But he chose not to.

Needles are at the epicentre of my life and will be until the day I die. In the nine months developing inside my mother's womb, one vital life-saving ingredient did not form: Factor VIII. Without it, my life would, at the very best, have involved decade upon decade of the internal bleeding that once caused me such profound, agonising pain as a toddler and young child. At worst, it would have killed me years ago, either from massive internal haemorrhaging or from infection with Hepatitis C or HIV. What has saved me from both those scenarios is the needles that inject synthetic Factor VIII into my body and allow me to live a normal life.

The medication makes me the same as anybody else. The training and dedication and sacrifice and hard work and willingness to go through pain make me an elite athlete. So, when a celebrated journalist who loves cycling has a choice of what needle to associate me with, I reserve the right to mark his homework. Because needles and I have a bit of history in a way that is totally different to any other professional cyclist on this earth.

My secondary school's attempt to educate my classmates about haemophilia was an archaic video where the key message was that a lot of haemophiliacs have HIV and hepatitis. Naturally, the reaction was a room full of children turning to stare at me and me having to say to them, 'Relax, it's not quite like that anymore. Thanks for your concern but I think that they need to update this video.'

In primary school, Wanda, the haemophiliac nurse (makes her sound like a superhero, which she is, really), gave Mum and Dad lessons in how to inject me. My parents would inject each other under Wanda's supervision as practice for the day they started injecting me. They fared well with each other, but I was a toddler, and if you look at a toddler's skin you can't see the veins, let alone feel them.

And as I have said, and he does not hide this, Dad found that he turned to jelly when he tried to put a needle in me. So, Mum did it and she carried a pager for the school to notify her if I had a bleed. It got plenty of use. At first, the pager was the cue to take me to hospital, and then, after she'd been trained, it meant she would come to school and give me my injection in the office of the headteacher, Mrs Mimpriss, after which I would return to class.

Once I was on prophylaxis, Mum would inject me three days a week before school. It was a long process because she'd have to put the numbing cream on my skin an hour beforehand. Sometimes she'd come in and do this while I was still asleep. Then she'd go down and get my Factor VIII from the fridge and mix its two component parts together. Just like the doctors and nurses, Mum couldn't always get the needle into a vein first time, so there were different places on my body she'd try. She was allowed to try twice – and if she couldn't find a vein with two attempts, then she'd take me into hospital.

It was not pleasant.

But it was a massive improvement on being rushed to hospital with a bleed, where the protocol was that the doctor or nurse was permitted four attempts to get the needle into my vein, and then, if they couldn't, a different medic would try. It was often three doctors, 12 attempts – 12 times a needle went into my skin – before they drew blood, and by then I was a mess and my parents were too.

Mum and Dad took it in turns to take me to hospital, to halve the number of times they went through the emotional shredder. As I cried and implored them to stop with the needles, my parents would soothe me but also have to ignore me, fixing their gaze on the needle going in and praying to see blood rise up through it.

The thing Mum found hardest – to the point that when I asked her to talk me through it for this book, she got very upset – was having her child look to her for protection and having instead to hold me down. I would often say:

'Mummy, I don't want this. Mummy, please, I don't want this.'

It killed a part of her every time.

They say that haemophiliacs grow up fast. Being taught how to inject yourself is a part of that. When the nurses decided I was ready to be taught how to self-inject, the thing I most wanted to know was if, at nine years of age, nearly 10, I was the youngest ever haemophiliac to be injecting myself. I was very competitive about it.

'Please can you find out?' I said to the nurse. 'Officially, am I the youngest?'

She did a very kind thing in leaving the room for two minutes and returning with confirmation that I was. True or not, I felt a million dollars.

I had to practice on my dad, that's how I learned. It was more traumatic for him than for me. A nurse would come to our house and teach us. It went well the first time I did it on myself. It was bound to, there was a world record at stake.

I never experienced any problems as a pro cyclist who has to inject himself. When joining a new team, I would pre-empt things by asking the team doctor to inform all the riders that they would see me injecting myself on race days with a non-performance-enhancing, blood-clotting agent. Most riders got told – though, as I've said, not all.

My routine on race days was to be given the plan of the day by the team, have breakfast, pack my stuff up, leave my suitcase outside my hotel room door and, if it was a Grand Tour, put my personal mattress and pillow outside my door as well, and go to the team bus. I would always board the bus early to take my medication, so as not to be putting a needle in my arm with the bus on the move.

There'd be another two lots of medication taken from the bus and put in the team car. The soigneurs or I would put them in the cool box with all of the bottles. Being in the team car, my medication was almost always behind me in the race and that's where you want it. If I crashed, then the medication would soon find me. Those scenarios in which I would be behind the team car were ones where the chances of me crashing were slim, because I would be out of the grupetto and not competitive. I would love to be able to tell you that situation never came to pass, but I can't.

The use of intravenous recovery was widespread in the generation of riders before mine. Most riders of my age, picking up the pieces of the sport after the doping era, have rejected all injections, including those of non-banned substances designed for post-stage recovery. The Movement for Credible Cycling, a union created to defend clean cycling, has 10 World Tour teams under its banner, including the team I have just spent the last three years of my World Tour career with, Israel Start-Up Nation. I never injected any recovery agents. I have only ever injected Factor VIII, which offers no help to performance at all other than the peace of mind of knowing you won't bleed to death if you crash today.

People might wince at the thought of a rider who injects every race day talking about recovery infusions and allegations of abusing TUEs (Therapeutic Use Exemptions), but why should I bow my head and look away, or be apologetically mute, when it comes to talking about this just because I rely on needles to keep me out of A&E and the morgue? As the only elite athlete in the world with haemophilia, I have more right than anyone to discuss and denounce needles and drug cheats. And I have more reason than anyone to bemoan teams that might have done nothing wrong but who, out of sheer arrogance, breed doubt and suspicion because they cannot produce medical records, and think they are bigger than the sport.

There is a story to write about me and drug-cheats, about me and needles. David Walsh's one-line version of it when covering my stage win in 2013 might have gone, 'Before yesterday, the 24-year-old was most famous for being the only haemophiliac in history to have become a professional cyclist' or he could have simply introduced me as the reigning British time trial champion (I had won the title two years running), but he chose to define me by my comment about Armstrong, uttered seven months earlier and withdrawn, explained and apologised for within hours.

I get that journalists need to define you in a few words and explain to their readers in shorthand who lesser-known figures like me are – I really don't need that explained to me – but I didn't understand the nugget of information David Walsh chose to select and define me by. I didn't understand why any journalist would look at my comments about Armstrong at the start line of a race and my immediate, unequivocal clarifications, look into my story and my career to date (looking into stuff is what journalists do, right?) and choose to write what he wrote. I didn't understand why he didn't stop and think, *Nah, he didn't know the full details of the USADA report at the time, he was about to race, he said something he would not have said two days later, he's made clear his position months ago, there's no good reason to bring that up again.*

As luck would have it, David Walsh was staying in the same hotel as I was the night he published his Stage 8 Giro piece. Except, it wasn't luck, because it was a team hotel and two teams were using it, Movistar and Team Sky, and I was a rider for Movistar and David Walsh was Team Sky's permanent guest. So, the chances of us running into each other weren't so slim.

David was sitting in reception. I went across to him and, because he had just won a journalism award, I said, 'I hear congratulations are in order.'

'Alex, no need for this,' he said.

'I mean it,' I said. 'Congratulations. Do you mind if I sit down?'

'Be my guest.'

'David, I want to tell you about that day in Beijing and how much we knew. I want to tell you about my history with Lance and where I was coming from.'

'You supported a guy that took drugs,' he said, with sparkling originality.

'Yes. At the time, I didn't know the full extent,' I said, 'but you've also got to understand that as a kid, this guy was most of our heroes and it's tough to accept that your heroes are not good people.'

We had a long conversation in which he never backed down on what he'd written. Instead, whilst I was feeling terribly down and hurt by it all, he issued what I guess was his version of a papal blessing in a series of Tweets saying nice things about me.

What I wished I'd had the presence of mind to say to him that evening, but I was too young and scared of his power to do so, and I knew I was no great debater, was that my stupid comment was seven months old when I won at the Giro and it would never have crossed my mind that he would choose to start a report on my first ever Grand Tour stage win by referencing that old comment.

The day after my Giro stage win, David Millar came looking for me, to congratulate me.

'Well done, Alex. That's huge. Really well done.'

'Thanks, David.'

'What's wrong?'

'Nothing.'

'You've just won your first Grand Tour race,' he said. 'You don't look like it. What's up?'

'Well, this guy, David Walsh, has written a real shitty thing about me and what I said in China.'

Millar's face dropped. He was fuming. He got straight onto Twitter and attacked Walsh. 'It's real disappointing that you've talked about your story, and not the story. One of the most significant moments in this guy's career, and you've chosen to use it as a platform for your own agenda.'

This was the perfect response to Walsh from the least ideal person. It was kind of David Millar and I felt profoundly supported by him, but he was a man with a history of drug-taking laying into the journalist who, second only to Paul Kimmage, was at the forefront of outing cycling's most prolific cheat. Cycling is a stupidly complicated beast, and with its drug history it ties itself up in knots. It's nice to be supported by someone when you are under attack, but I loathe cheating and I don't think cheats should be allowed to race and David Millar falls into that category.

I know that might come across as ungrateful, but I've earned the right to talk about fairness and cheating, not simply because I am clean – that really isn't and shouldn't be a claim to fame any more – but because I have always measured myself against athletes who do not have a rare disease. I have never used my condition for gain and plenty of people don't even know that there is no other haemophiliac in elite, professional world sport.

I'm a firm believer in lifetime bans. If a case is black and white, like David Millar's owning up was, I don't believe in second chances within sport. Second chances in life? Absolutely. Second, third, fourth chances, you never give up on someone. But when you cheat everyone else in your sport, the cost for other competitors is devastating. For the person who gets sent a Gold medal in the post by the Olympic Committee eight years after he or she got a Silver, it is meaningless and devastating.

I think 99% of cyclists operate within the rules. I think that abuse of the very necessary TUE falls into the grey, a fact that is profoundly unfair on all riders, and especially those with genuine illnesses or conditions which require medication.

Without cheating Lance Armstrong was average. He got a disease and he came back a cheat. He used his illness to win sympathy and support and admiration and he lied to the community of cancer sufferers, a community of people for whom hope is like oxygen or water. That is unforgiveable.

Yes, for a while Armstrong was a legend. But he turned out to be the worst possible role model for children. I want children with haemophilia to hear me and transform their view of their own life. To think, 'Yes, I can do that. I can move more, do more, live more.' I've given my life to cycling and I've put myself through pain and seclusion and mental torture to do it. That's why, despite how he portrayed me, I admire David Walsh, who put himself through so much to uncover the truth – a truth that serves cycling well, perhaps even saved it.

David has talked about the most upsetting aspect to his investigation being the riders and soigneurs who Lance Armstrong trashed and bullied and, in some cases, crushed. He has said he was motivated less by going after Armstrong and more by standing up for them. How extraordinary of him, then, to go for me the way he did seven months after I'd made a mistake and set the record straight.

11

GROWING UP

On the Road with Cavendish, 2013–2015

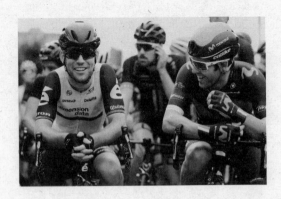

If I had to sum up the first half of my five years at Movistar, I would say that winning bike races, driving a flash car and earning a lot of money was what defined me.

It was a great time to be a part of Movistar. My Stage 8 Giro win was just one of 32 stage wins for the team in 2013, which saw us finish the World Tour in the number one spot. Team Sky were second. Nairo Quintana came second in the Tour de France, where he and Rui Costa secured three stage wins between them for the team. I won the National Time Trial Championships for the third successive year.

But despite the success, I seemed to be working my way through too many coaches and wasn't happy with my training. The team were used to Spanish riders who lived in the mountains and trained a certain way. I was being asked to go on four-hour hikes in my off season. It was so far removed from what I was used to that it unnerved me. I failed to click with two of Movistar's leading coaches, Xabier Artetxe and Mikel Zabala, both hugely talented but not what I needed as a TT specialist. I wasn't open-minded, not enough to swap bike training for rambling. I never heard of Wiggins going for walks.

Things weren't meshing. Movistar were pushing me to develop my hill climbing, but anybody who looked at my power output, weight and physique knew I was no mountain goat. I was being put into events where I didn't stand a chance of doing well and then felt criticised for my performance. And, believe me, even when Movistar weren't critical, I was heavily self-critical.

To get myself back on track, I turned to the Maldon 10 on my doorstep in Essex. It was the first time trial I had ever done as a boy, the one that qualified me for the George Herbert Stancer Memorial National Youth Time Trial Championship in 2003, where competitive cycling grabbed hold of me and changed my life. I knew that I trained well on that route and was still working on trying to crack 18 minutes there. In the grand scheme of things, it might seem like an insignificant pin on the cycling map, but the Maldon 10 was the environment in which I addressed the fact that I never really had much more power to play with as a cyclist. I worked on making up for that power deficit by mixing up pacing strategies, working out what to do with the wind, when to push on in a tailwind or when to ease off. I made mistakes and I gained knowledge there. Michael Hutchinson called it my laboratory.

The lanes of rural Essex take you across a treasure trove of beautiful, calm flatlands that are, I am pleased to report, largely ignored or unknown. Farmland peppered with small villages, thatched cottages, windmills and streams, rolls gently towards the Suffolk border. I have ridden this landscape with many cyclists, some of whom have won multiple stages of the Tour de France and some you will never have heard of. I have learned from all of them equally, no matter their fame.

Andy Lyons is one of my oldest mates, in both senses of the word; I've known him since I was a teenager and he's as old as the hills that Essex does not possess. He was an elite cyclist in the UK for 25 years, rode for GB and did a handful of World Tour races, and so not only did he understand the level I was riding at, he had a shedload of experience racing bikes. I don't know half of what Andy knows:

he's not had the career I've had, but he's been able to enjoy racing a bike as a lone amateur, riding on instinct, not providing leadouts and tactical deliveries for other riders like I have, always racing to win. He knows plenty that pro tour riders don't understand. I have always sought his opinion and the hundreds of five-hour training rides we've notched up have been the place I've done it.

We'd normally head to North Essex and into Suffolk, sometimes Herts. There were no conditions we wouldn't go out in. Andy mentored me as a youngster and then, when I turned pro, he would never want me to knock a single kilometre off my training to stay with him, so he'd push and push himself and wreck himself doing it. I owe him a great deal.

Mark Cavendish lives in Essex and, for a couple of years, he regularly joined Andy and me on our training runs. Horribly successful, revoltingly talented, Cav has a roll of honour proclaiming him one of the greatest and most unique talents in road race history. When we first started riding together on the Essex lanes in 2013, he had just won five stages of the Giro, either side of my one, on his way to winning the green jersey. His triumph on Stage 12 was his 100th professional win. The year before, he had become the most successful sprinter in the history of the Tour de France.

No wonder he came looking to me for help.

Our training runs were phenomenal. We pushed each other hard and I didn't blow smoke up his backside. In return, his towering standards created a day-to-day normality in the saddle which offered me the chance to improve. I observed him, quarried for wisdom when he was up for talking, and let him be when he was not. It's impossible to measure the boost that training alongside someone that good gives you. You stop thinking and get on with the work instead, and your levels go up and immediately feel normal. For someone like me, who can overthink things, reducing training down to the simple goal of being good enough to ride with Mark Cavendish and also be of some use to him was a welcome respite from the confused state of my coaching at Movistar.

Cav, Andy and I trained extremely hard together and got the best out of each other. On one session we were murdering each other, pushing and goading without respite for 70km before stopping, as we often did, at the Blue Egg Cafe. As we parked up, I noticed Andy was glaring at me.

'What's up?' I said.

'When we're tearing into you out there,' he said, 'you became a different person. A killer. If you rode like that on the tour, if you were less nice, you'd win more races.'

He marched off into the café. I turned and saw Cav smiling to himself and nodding.

Andy and I have covered tens of thousands of East Anglian miles together and I've learned more from him than every team coach in my career added together. When I talk about the greats of cycling, I include Andy Lyons among them. His one fault was that he never stopped moaning about how my lack of mudguards meant I would spray and splash him in the slipstream. I had an image to maintain and was not about to put mudguards on a £10,000 bike. Eventually, however, he banged on about it so much one winter that I decided I'd rather be the only World Tour rider with mudguards than listen to Andy Lyons complain about it for another second.

I felt like an idiot and my bike looked like a tractor.

After the Giro Stage victory, I started getting emails from parents of haemophiliac children saying that seeing someone with the disease on the World Tour was making them question the restrictions on their own child's life. I wondered for the first time if my disease was something I could be proud of, rather than downplaying it for fear of being uninvited to the ultimate party – the UCI World Tour.

I got involved in an awareness-raising campaign called Miles for Haemophilia, which involved me travelling around Europe and to the US to advocate for healthy, active lifestyles for haemophiliacs, and talk about my experiences.

I knew that I wanted to do something useful, but I was also being paid to do these talks. I have to be straight in saying that, back then, I would not have done these talks for free.

What I discovered quickly was the impact my story made. I talked about the expectations I began my life with – of wheelchairs, crutches, joints fused in place – to a room full of people living with exactly these same prospects for their children. Hearing how I lived confounded their worse expectations. It gave them hope.

I also realised that telling them about my parents was just as inspirational as talking about my career, and more relevant. I told people all across Europe about how Mum and Dad had sidestepped the negativity and managed my haemophilia so that I lived normally.

'But being an elite athlete isn't normal,' people would say.

'But growing up with a right to dream and have goals and work hard to achieve them is normal. It doesn't matter what the specific goal is. It's about equal opportunity to have a full life.'

I told audiences that I had set my personal best speed on the Tour of Switzerland that same year at 118km/h (73mph). 'You can see why my mum worries,' I said. 'The point is that my career isn't without worry and risk, but haemophiliacs can assess and take risk like other people, rather than just pull up the drawbridge on their needs and ambitions.'

Gradually, I honed my message so that I could be as useful as possible for the campaign. But no such refinement existed in my own life. I was still immature and not getting my head around being paid plenty of money. My salary had been on an upward arc from Trek-Livestrong to Sky and Movistar and I presumed it would keep going up as I got better. And while I knew that an elite cyclist's career is a very short one and the money needs to last a long time, the trajectory of my pay packet told me one thing: *I must be really good at this*.

I should have realised that I needed to keep developing myself, that training hard on my own terrain and handpicking coaches was not the path to glory. I should have been asking more questions and focusing on what the riders ahead of me were doing. And the thing is, I am fairly polite and well-behaved and quiet, so it's not as if I was acting like a massive tosser on a grand enough scale for my team, family or friends to get alarmed and rein me in. I was just quietly, politely waiting for greatness to come to me and going about things with a bit of an attitude. And I would continue to do so until I met my future wife and she kicked the stuffing right out of me.

And it was not as if I was misfiring in a struggling team. In 2014, Movistar again won the World Tour. Nairo Quintana won the Giro d'Italia. Alejandro Valverde was world number one and Movistar described me as one of their outstanding youngsters, for my contribution to the team throughout the season and my Gold at the Commonwealth Games in Glasgow.

I was doing well enough on the bike that I did not feel compelled to change myself, nor did I feel the need to improve things radically. And I had this fear of missing out, implanted in me as a kid. All my mates had gone off to university, and I was itching for some of those experiences and went after some good times that might imitate them. I wanted to meet women I wanted to party with my mates. I did a stupid amount of go-karting because I had a bunch of mates who all loved it and were all quick.

Movistar wanted me to move to Spain, to train in hot weather and at altitude, to be more a part of the team. I was worried about moving away from the NHS, but that was not the main reason I stayed in England. I wanted a good time and that wasn't going to happen up a mountain; neither was any of the other fun I was finally having.

Professionally I was thinking that the way I was doing things was working in many respects, and that if I went and did the same as everyone else at Movistar, I would be the same as everyone else. Movistar had employed me to be the time trialist and someone good on the flat. They had an abundance of guys that climbed mountains well.

If I get 20% better at going uphill, I'm still not winning the Tour de France or anything that involves inclines.

I felt a certain defiance about this: *Let me be the rider I think you employed me to be.*

With hindsight, I think they employed me thinking I was going to be someone who could get up a hill better than I do. But Movistar never really pressured you to do anything. It was all done on a suggestion basis. *We think you should do this to be better*, but that was the extent of their development. *You should eat less and you should move somewhere hilly.*

Me thinking I knew better, and Movistar being laid-back about making me change, was mixed with another pretty unhelpful ingredient: my obsession with fast cars. I was spending too much time and far too much money on them. Dad liked them, naturally. He's an ex-racing driver, so it would have been strange if he hadn't.

My Lotus Exige SV6 was 380bhp, but very light, and went like a rocket. I sold it because one morning I found myself sat behind a pick-up truck realising I was head height to its towbar.

If I get it all wrong in this car, I'll be dead, I realised.

I had decided that when I got picked for the 2014 Tour de France I would get myself a Mercedes C Class Black series as a present to myself. It was crazy money and the only upside of not getting selected was being saved from making that mistake. Instead, I made a different mistake, being duped out of thousands of pounds buying a Mercedes AMG SUV from a con artist who preyed on athletes saying he could source great deals for sports stars from elite car brands. It was a big loss, financially, but I loved the car. I followed it up with the best car I've ever had, a Mercedes C63 Edition 1, matt grey with the yellow stripe. That thing was wild. I loved it and even sold it at a profit, despite driving it out of the showroom and rinsing it for a year. It was a small win, one marginal gain among a litany of four-wheel losses, and gave me a taste for cars that made money. So, I got a 10-year-old 911 GT3. It was raw and manual and had an old radio and was a great fun, even though it scared me shitless.

Mum wasn't happy about the cars at all. She didn't like them and she was appalled by my spending on them. I bought her a Mercedes SLC to address that issue. I bought my sister a car too, the Fiat 500 Abarth, a great little hot hatch. Lois had a heart attack when she went to insure it. (I didn't think that through.) I bought my mum two handbags that she'd always wanted as well. It's nice to be able to do those things, but who was I doing it for? For Mum? Or for me to feel good about myself and to look good? There was plenty of the latter going on. I was cocky, loyal and loving, and in denial. If your mum wants a serious conversation with you about your lifestyle and you don't want to hear it, then buying her a car is a good way to put her on the back foot.

I didn't spend money on Dad, just supplied him with free kit from sponsors. I won a bike for winning the National Road Race Series and had it customised for him. I think he liked that.

There was a bit of me thinking, *I'm doing this because I owe them everything for giving me the life I have*. The truth, as any parent will tell you, is they don't want thanks. But more than that, if I really was going to thank my parents for what they've given me and done for me, then a car, a handbag, a bike – well, it's pathetic.

———

I travelled out to Lisbon for the Global Summit on Haemophilia and Dan Hart was there beside me. We did a joint presentation and, at the Q&A, a doctor in the audience stood up and said,

'I think what you do is deeply irresponsible. Selfish and irresponsible. Every single facet of what you have said today is irresponsible. It sets a bad example to the health system and it's expensive.'

The room went quiet. My brain went blank.

I had done a few of these events by now and seen some lovely cities and been put up in nice hotels and, frankly, I had been told I was inspirational and amazing by a host of different people. But as I sat in that room in Lisbon, in silence, with the doctor waiting for a reply, I was out of my depth.

I'd never been on the receiving end of this specific criticism before, which is not to say I hadn't considered it. In fact, I had often asked myself if I was doing the right thing, going from country to country encouraging haemophiliacs to get active? And it is obviously true that if I was not a pro cyclist I would not have broken as many bones as I have and used up the resources I did. On top of that is the responsibility I have to take for causing worry. My career does upset Lois and my mum because there's a risk. Lois took me aside when she was young and I was at the Academy and said she didn't want me to die. Dad worries when things go wrong. Mum worries all the time. I have put them through a lot in choosing to race bikes at the top level.

I know that on race days Mum often finds herself sitting around the house, distracted, staring out the window, a bit lost. She's worrying. That's her unfair return for being brave enough to allow me to race bikes instead of working in an office. I live this exciting life, loads of travel, lots of challenges, occasional success and adulation, and she's left holding a mug of tea, staring out the window and telling herself not to imagine me lying lifeless on the road.

Dad waits for his phone to ring on race days. If the call comes around 4 p.m. or after, it's from me. If it comes early afternoon, he knows it's a crash. I have sometimes thought about it, on the start line. *This race finishes in five hours' time. Am I going to be in an ambulance or on the podium?*

Of course, as a leadout man and time trialist, the reality is usually neither.

But that particular set of concerns has nothing to do with haemophilia and everything to do with crashing. The doctor at the Lisbon talk was raising an important question but had been so direct about it, so cold and unequivocal, that I didn't know what to say. I had experience only of talking to a benign audience.

Dan Hart stepped in.

'Let's look at this from another point of view,' he said. 'If Alex wasn't a pro cyclist, he'd probably be 15–20 kilos heavier and require 2,500 or 3,000 units of medication every other day instead of the 2,000 that he takes, because Factor VIII dosage is based on weight. So that's one bigger cost, for starters. And there'd also be more strain on his muscles and joints, they'd be weaker, so he'd also probably have a lot more bleeding episodes. I wouldn't mind betting that Alex as a pro cyclist, despite the broken bones, is less of a drain on the health care system than Alex as a regular citizen.'

The doctor nodded and sat down. I respected her for making an important challenge in front of a crowd who were very pro me and on board with our message. She didn't make herself popular, but she got everyone thinking, me included. What was great was that Dan's answer really made everyone in the room think too. He moved the ideas we were putting forward on to another level. We looked at what he had said, which all stacked up – of course it did – and this pragmatic, economic, vindication of haemophiliacs being more active, living more, moving more, would one day become the founding principle for my charity.

The training rides with Cav in Essex petered out. I'm not sure why. People ask me if I fell out with him, because we seemed to be in each other's lives and then not. The answer is, not that I'm aware of. On some days, Cav just did not want to talk and I would ask myself, *Have I done something wrong?* I felt privileged to have Mark Cavendish to train with on a regular basis, but I was never relaxed with him. I was in awe of him and struggled to be myself. But that came from me, not him. It's something I didn't like about myself. Cav and his wife, Peta, invited me to stay with them in Italy before my Hour record attempt in 2015 while I recovered from the shoulder blade injury. I always felt more comfortable talking to Peta than I did to Mark. What he wanted was some company on the roads. I tried to give him that, to judge as best as I could when he wanted to talk and when he didn't. I've no idea when I got that right or wrong, but I have no regrets because riding with him those two years in Essex was one of the greatest experiences of my life.

What I admire about Cav is that he is a racer, no matter what. I probably wouldn't contest a bunch sprint, but he would always contest a time trial, unless it was really long and in a Grand Tour. After Team Sky had a poor Tour of Britain in 2012, he and I raced at an event on London's Embankment. Geraint Thomas was Sky's main contender to win it and he crashed. I won the morning time trial on the embankment and that lifted the mood of Sean Yates and the management. In the afternoon, Cav won the criterium.

'Mate, I don't know how you do it,' I told him. 'I was next to you with a kilometre to go and I just wasn't physically good enough to even maintain position. As the speed went up, you flew through all that.'

He just shrugged. 'Yeah, and in the morning, I went as hard as I could in that time trial and you were pulling three seconds per kilometre out of me. I do not understand how.'

I've never forgotten that, in part because it was Mark Cavendish being incredibly generous about me, but mainly because it encapsulated what many people don't understand about cycling, the way it has radically different disciplines within the same race. You don't see Usain Bolt and Eliud Kipchoge on the same start line or being compared for their performances relative to each other.

Cav was interested in why I was good in a TT, but he wasn't threatened. He didn't see it as competition. He was happy for me. I was in awe of him, I still am, but he was reminding me that we do very different things. That's what confuses people about cycling and leader boards; whereas in track different types of athletes (sprinters, distance runners) do not line up in the same race, in cycling there's a bunch of different types of athlete lining up for the same race with totally different given jobs to do and criteria for success. That rider who appears DNF or 180th in a race result, and who ran the leadout that set up a team victory, is the most valuable member of a cycling team that day and paid highly for his role. But on paper he's an also-ran at best, a total loser at worst.

What Cav has to endure has been rough at times. The first year that he didn't win five stages of the Tour de France (and he still won some) he had sponsors asking, 'What went wrong?' That's got to be hard. Cav lives at that level of expectation where anything less than a win in the highest echelon of sport is deemed a failure. He divides opinion and that's part and parcel of sprinting and the persona you have to carry with it, but the criticism he has received has been colossal and often ignorant. I've received criticism, but it's been minute in comparison, because my achievements are small in comparison to his.

In Mum and Dad's downstairs WC is a massive photo of me on the track with Cavendish. It was taken at a time when I was in very good shape and Cav was coming back from injury and was visibly struggling. Cav is on my wheel and looks in trouble, trailing in my wake, and in that respect the photograph captures a very rare moment indeed. My parents had it enlarged and hung above the toilet, so if you go for a pee at their house, that's what's looking back at you.

A legend. And Alex Dowsett.

———

Another month, another European city on the Miles for Haemophilia campaign. In Barcelona, a mother asked me, through a translator, 'What would your team do if you crashed?'

'It's not *if*,' I replied. 'It's *when*. If I can get up and carry on, I will. If I can't, then the medication is in the car and I either take some or go to hospital to be checked out.'

'Oh,' she said, 'so not much different to anyone else on the team, really?'

'No difference. The hospital will see the medication and know what to do.'

'But if you are in a high-risk sport and your team treats you no differently, why should my son be treated differently at school?'

'He shouldn't be.'

After the event, I was talking to a small group of people and became aware of the mother coming towards me. She was pulling the translator with her by the arm. I turned away from the group and smiled at her. And as I reached out to shake her hand, I saw that she was tearful. She didn't shake my hand. She put her arms around me and hugged me. She was shaking.

'I am going to change my son's life,' she said.

I think this was the moment my charity was conceived.

Bike races are great, winning them is one of the best feelings I know. But what she made me feel will never leave me. I had given her the impetus to change her son's life, but I knew that she would not necessarily find the resources and mentality back home to support her. I know what is needed to transform the life of haemophiliacs. Doing something with my knowledge was no longer a nagging idea. It was a responsibility.

It was time to up the ante on my training. I knew that Movistar were too laid-back with me, possibly because they weren't sure what to do with me, so it was down to me to stop complaining and do something. One of the things I turned to was the idea of epically fast motor pacing sessions and it was brilliant. It did a lot for my speed.

Motor pacing is when you train by riding your bike behind a motorbike at high speed for a long time. To do it you need a motorbike and mates like I had in Jack and Liam. I decided to go for 48+ km/h averages over rides of between 145–160km. No easing off. Laughably, we had a knackered, pale blue, unsightly moped rather than a motorbike and looked like the Del Boy and Rodney Trotter of the motor pacing world. We not only looked ridiculous but sounded it too, with a 50cc engine tuned to its limits. I had to use earplugs.

In reality, the moped was perfect. You don't want a twitchy, powerful motorbike struggling to stay down at 30mph. The moped was more like a relentlessly fit and fast cyclist, a tireless, robotic version of the toughest opposition you could possibly face. We'd leave at 6 or 7 a.m. and have the roads to ourselves, mostly pan flat but there were some rollers, and neither Jack or Liam would slow down for them, so where I would normally spend 30–40 seconds on these little climbs doing 300 watts, when motor pacing I'd spend 10–15 seconds on them doing 800 watts, just to keep up. Jack had a particularly fine feel for getting me on the absolute limit and keeping me there. Both he and Liam were friends from very early days and I was incredibly lucky that they both would happily sit on that old moped for two or three hours at a time. They seemed to enjoy it. I don't know why. We'd end up at the Blue Egg Café as a resting and refuelling stop about three-quarters of the way through a 100-mile effort. One day, at the next table, there was a guy I knew by sight. He was an avid cyclist but not a racer.

He said, 'How much have you done?'

When someone asks you that before saying hello you know what sort of chat is incoming.

'Oh, 70 miles so far, I think.'

'Behind a moped it's easy, isn't it?'

'Yes, it's easy,' I said. 'Tell you what, jump on for the way back, because we're all going in the same direction. See if you enjoy it.'

He lasted 200m. He literally disappeared from view with the café still in sight. I had, admittedly, said to Jack, 'No mercy' as we started.

Another time an elderly woman followed us in her car for 20 miles. There were few chances for her to overtake, but she didn't seem to be trying. She stayed right on my tail until we got to a junction where we had to stop and she pulled up next to us. We braced ourselves for some criticism and, sure enough, her window went down.

'I don't know anything about cycling, but I've been sat behind you for miles and that was brilliant. You're amazing. Well done.'

It put a smile on my face that even Jack and his 50cc of brute power couldn't wipe off.

You can't replicate the peloton in training, but motor pacing can get you used to doing whatever it takes to stay with the pace. If a coach asked me to do 15 seconds at 800 watts, I would politely suggest it wasn't a great idea. When you're chasing your mate on a motorbike, you're not even looking at the power. You're simply doing what's needed to keep up and that is sometimes what racing is.

A few years later, in the build-up to the 2019 Tour de France, I would have conversations with my coaches at Team Katusha–Alpecin and beg them to stop obsessing about the wattage and concentrate on racing. Motor pacing gets your brain used to the idea of sticking with a pace and fighting to be up there, of speed not power – because when it comes to racing, the fastest crosses the finish line first, not the most powerful. Indeed, it is rarely the most powerful.

I had raced as part of the great Team Sky. I had spent a formative year leaning from the peerless Taylor Phinney. My team, Movistar, were winners of the World Tour in 2013, 2014 and 2015 and I spent hundreds of hours in the wind tunnel. But Essex is where the lion's share of what made me a successful bike rider took place.

I trained bloody hard – not just the motor pacing, everything – but I found I was going back to the same races and knocking out the same results. That's why my interest in learning about aerodynamics and skin suits and bike tech and all the gains to be made in the minutiae became an obsession. (Dave Brailsford had always been way ahead of the curve on all of this.)

I asked Movistar repeatedly for changes that they wouldn't, or couldn't, allow because of sponsorship deals. Again and again, I lobbied for us to be able to use the Osymetric chainrings I'd had at Sky, to maximise the effectiveness of the dead spot in the pedalling action and engage the hamstrings and glutes more, but I got nowhere. Campagnolo wouldn't let it happen and Movistar were hugely dictated to by their sponsors. After three years there, in November 2015, I sat down with Eusebio in Pamplona and raised the subject again.

'Why do you keep asking for these chain rings, Alex? No one who is good likes them.'

'Except Chris Froome, the guy who just won the Tour de France.'

Eusebio paused, then laughed. 'Okay. It's still no.'

We both knew it was about sponsors, but it was hard to get too annoyed at Eusebio. He lives and breathes cycling and his boundless energy has made him the longest-running team manager on the World Tour. He is a survivor and one of his secrets is giving sponsors the same importance as winning races, and he is a man who has strong, sound values.

It was Eusebio who jumped on board with my ambition to have a crack at the Hour and helped make that happen in 2015. He understood fully and supported my growing belief that the Hour record being held by a haemophiliac could lead to a whole lot of good things for other people with the disease. The Olympics and Commonwealths, and the Tour de France, mean something to some people, but everyone understands a world record. I couldn't guarantee a Gold at Rio in 2016 and I was not going to win the Tour de France unless they swapped the mountain stages for time trials in Holland and Belgium, but I had long had my eyes set on the Hour record.

When I told Eusebio that my experiences of meeting the parents of haemophiliacs across Europe had added another reason to have a crack at it and to train myself into the ground to succeed, he threw Movistar behind it – and the result was that fantastic day in Manchester on which we took the Hour record and began, I hope, to inspire people with rare diseases to do more, move more, and transform their lives.

I am proud of the fact that in Movistar's own team history they have put my Hour record up there as a defining part of yet another outstanding year for us as a team. We were, once again, winners of the World Tour. Nairo Quintana and Alejandro Valverde were exceptional all year, mind-blowing at times. Their second and third overall in the Tour de France, my first Tour, saw Movistar finish first in the teams' classification in a great collective performance. Marc Soler announced his arrival at the top level by winning the Tour de l'Avenir. I won the National Time Trial Championships for the fourth time in five years, meaning that Movistar was home to the national TT champions of GB, Italy and Spain.

So, by the late spring of 2015 I was an integral part of the best team in world cycling, holder of the Hour record, showing the first signs of abandoning my idiot-car-buying policy and my ideas for a Haemophilia charity were beginning to take shape.

I thought life could not get better and that I was all grown up, but I was about to be proved wrong on both counts.

12

MUMMY'S BOY

It's All About Love, 2016

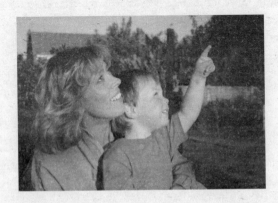

They say that elite athletes can put themselves through suffering other people can't comprehend. In the autumn of 2016 and early winter of 2017, I withstood levels of indifference and the brush-off from a woman called Chanel Harris which far outweighed any previous test of my endurance.

2016 was a topsy-turvy year. I put in performances ranging from the average to the good (at the Tour of Dubai, Vuelta a Castilla y León and Tour de Suisse) to the very good (a fourth in the TT at Tirreno–Adriatico, after a brilliant battle with Cancellara, Johan Le Bon and Tony Martin). The poor days reminded me I had plenty to improve on, the good ones that I could win on any given day and that the Giro was there for me to take by the horns. I was crowned National TT champion for the fifth time, won the TT at the Tour of Poland and watched the first serious relationship that I'd ever had hit the rocks. We fell in love quickly, but with me always putting the bike first, it fell apart equally as fast.

It was also the year of the Giro that got away, something that still drives me crazy more than half a decade later. The time trials at that year's Giro were just right for me. I was eyeing up the prospect of wearing a career-defining pink jersey on the start line of Stage 2 if I won a prologue that was technical and short, and suited me perfectly. The bike, bars and suit were fast. Our front wheel was the only weakness in our set-up; the only place we gave anything away.

Two weeks out from the Giro, I noticed a patch of skin on my collarbone change colour, where it had been plated the year before. The next day, a hole appeared in my skin. I looked closely and I could see the metal plate. Livio di Mascio, the surgeon at the Royal London, took a look.

'We need to take that plate out, but it's very straightforward, a 25-minute surgery.'

'Cool. I can still do the Giro.'

He narrowed his eyes. 'The Giro's gone, Alex.'

'Wha…'

'That plate has to come out today before infection and there's a lot of screw holes in your collarbone. It's going to take six weeks for those to calcify. That's a very weak collarbone you've got there. If you fall, it'll break.'

I was horrified. 'Yes, but I could fall off in training.'

'Which is why you won't be training.'

I watched the prologue – and that was probably a bad idea. The Dutch rider Tom Dumoulin won it in the sort of time I had been knocking out all year. It was the same scenario in the main TT on Stage 9. Cancellara was sick and way off the pace in fourth. Stefan Küng, Jos van Emden, all the hitters, fell away. An up-and-coming Primož Roglič won and I was confident it would have been mine given my form.

I was devastated. It felt like the biggest missed opportunity of my career. There were no positives to take from it. I didn't even have the luxury of being able to pop down the Alex Dowsett wormhole and blame myself. I hadn't crashed. I hadn't done anything stupid. That would have been better. I'm always more than happy when I can lay into myself. It was just bad luck. When I was allowed back in the saddle, I went home to the Maldon 10 and promptly smashed the TT record there with a time of 19.08 at an average of 50 km/h, and the following week won the Nationals.

The only way to deal with something like that is to tell yourself that these things balance themselves out; that I've won races when a rival punctured or was absent through injury. But the 2016 Giro was such a huge lost opportunity for a pink jersey and, I believe, two stage wins, that I've always taken the other option with this one: I remain permanently pissed off and inconsolable.

With my first proper relationship and the Grand Tour I also loved both gone, it was time to do something constructive. So, I sought solace by tearing my way through Tinder. One fateful day, a woman called Chanel popped up. I swiped right, we matched and started 'talking'. It was hard work from my point of view, with my persistence being met with her indifference. I asked her out on more than one occasion and, when she finally agreed to meet up, she bailed on me.

Not hellbent on retaining any dignity, I watched this same thing – me ask her out, her agree, her pull out – happen multiple times.

I mean, I was a professional athlete with two highly photogenic kittens. Why was this happening? I thought I'd covered all my bases.

Chanel lived in Balham, along with half the global population of Kiwis and Australians. She loved London and had never ventured beyond the M25 because she was too busy living what she calls *her very best single life*, having a lot of fun after moving to the UK at the end of a long-term relationship in New Zealand. She'd been on Tinder for over a year and it was not somewhere she expected to find long-term love.

Shopping for men on the internet, she called it.

I sent her a series of messages in late 2016: Happy Birthday, Happy Christmas, Happy New Year. None of them got a response. Thin-skinned as I am on the bike, I seemed to be thick-skinned to the point of stupidity off it. In early January I sent Chanel a message: *You play hard to get really well. This is my last try before I delete you, but do you want to go for that drink on Wednesday night? I promise you won't regret it.*

Unfathomably, given her radio silence for the preceding month, she replied, 'Yes'. Not to a drink on Wednesday, though. She'd do lunch on Saturday, when she had nothing better on.

I have never once been on the front foot with her.

We had one person in common. Chanel knew the girlfriend of George Bennett, the New Zealand cyclist making a name for himself at Team Jumbo-Visma. George already had a reputation for being an outstanding team player on the bike and a genuine bloke off it, and was on the cusp of his first pro GC victory at the Tour of California.

Professional athletes travelling the world don't have the greatest reputation when it comes to being faithful to their partners and cycling is no exception. George had told Chanel stories about riders being arseholes. Chanel messaged George to find out if I was one of them. He replied that, as far as he knew, I wasn't.

I wish he'd been right about that.

For our much anticipated (by me) and often cancelled (by her) first date, I wore red corduroy trousers and a jacket and scarf – a dapper, English Gent look with a cheeky Essex twist.

'Wow, that's a bold move for a first date,' she said.

Literally the first words out of her mouth.

It was more of an interview than a date. She bombarded me with questions and paid for lunch. I didn't know what had hit me. We met at Jamie's Italian in Stratford. I had gallantly suggested the location as a midway point and it was only then that she clocked I didn't live in London.

'Where *do* you live then?'

'Have you heard of Essex?'

'Yeah, sure.'

'There.'

'Where is it? I've heard of it, no idea where it is.'

'Not far,' I said, a bit too desperately. 'Just on from Northeast London. A town called Chelmsford.'

'Oh, cool. What's it like?'

'Er, I dunno. Hard to pick out a favourite aspect, really. I like it.'

'I feel like I'm there.'

I decided not to mention that, had I offered to come into central London to meet her, it would have affected my training schedule – and I never let anything do that.

I had a salad and she had a salad. She wasn't drinking in January and I wasn't drinking full stop.

'A very wholesome date,' she muttered.

I laughed, 'Yeah, look at us.' And I asked her what she normally did for first dates.

'Bars,' she said. 'Always bars and alcohol.' She'd been on a date the evening before and had one the next day. In turn, she was the fourth person I had taken to Jamie's Italian that week.

We deserved each other.

Chanel worked for a marketing firm and advertising agency in London. She had no idea about cycling, thought I was a courier and that the Tour de France was a one-day race. When I explained it wasn't, she asked me if I'd ever won it.

'No.'

'Were you at the Olympics, in London?'

'No. You mean as a competitor or a spectator?'

'Competitor.'

'No.'

'Oh. Spectator?'

'No.'

'Oh.'

The Q&A continued. I started mixing my answers up a bit, throwing in a yes here and there. At one point, I used the salt and pepper shakers to explain what a slipstream is, because that always sets hearts racing.

'And you're paid to do this?' she said.

'Yes, I'm paid. It's my job.'

'That's cool. It doesn't sound like you win much. How are you being paid?'

'Well, often, I'm working for someone else in a race.'

She realised quickly that she was getting to know somebody who was probably going to 'lose' virtually every race he entered. Not only that, but he would often be heaped with praise for doing so because he was setting someone else up to win the race. She considered this an interesting professional dynamic, which might require therapy in the long term.

'You must have to have a really good mentality to know that every time you get on that start line, you know your percentage of winning is so tiny. You must go insane when you do win.'

'I do actually, yeah,' I said. 'I tend to either go numb or behave like an idiot.'

I resisted telling her I was a five-time National Champion and had broken the Hour record – for two reasons. Firstly, I needed something in reserve for a second date, should that occur. Second up, the prospect of describing the Hour record to someone who found even a normal bike race so ridiculous was not looking good.

I could see her picking up the salt shaker and just twirling it round in circles. 'You do this?'

We would have more conversations in the months and years that followed about the psychology of being a professional bike rider. Fiercely intelligent, logical and kind, Chanel would tell me one day that I should be mindful of what a headfuck it is to be invited to go pro in a sport because you are winning lots of races, only for your job to become setting others up to win races. I would soon need all her counsel and wisdom on this subject when I rode for Katusha in the service of Marcel Kittel, but I'll come to that later.

After our date we exchanged a few messages that turned into more messages, and then a couple of phone calls, and then we had a period when I was abroad racing and we were messaging each other all day when I wasn't on the bike, often within seconds of getting off it. I would call her most evenings and we'd easily, happily, spend two or three hours chatting and getting to know each other. For the first time in my life, I was out on my bike thinking of someone other than myself and of something other than the bike. And I was missing someone I hardly knew.

When I got back, Chanel took me to Ottolenghi restaurant on a date and, God, it was awful. I was so hungry. I had come off a big day's training and looked at these tiny portions of photogenic nothingness and knew I just couldn't order 30 of them to make up a normal-sized recovery meal without scaring her off and bankrupting her.

That ordeal behind me, we entered that extraordinary part of a relationship where we learned about each other and each other's lives. Or at least that's how it was to me. I was loving spending time with her, fitting it in around my job as a cyclist and not giving it all too much thought. But Chanel was trying to get her head around how much cycling impacted everything in my life and beginning to see parts of me she didn't really like. But she gave me the benefit of the doubt.

We were in a relationship, but we weren't. We were talking a lot, but mostly only meeting up when Chanel could come out to see me in Essex. I showed her the delights of Essex's finest beach. Chanel and her friend were thoroughly unimpressed.

Frinton-on-Sea. Another trump card from the pack played to no effect.

—————

Athletes are selfish. We live in fear of diluting our commitment to our training even fractionally and losing as a result. My job is not a 35 hours per week affair. It's a 24/7 life sentence to being as good as you can before they cart you off to the knacker's yard. It takes a pretty special partner to understand that and even then there's no reason why they would choose it.

I was saying all the right things, but not actually doing anything differently. I imagine I thought I was, but in fact, without noticing it, I hadn't changed at all. Tareq, some friends and I were having a party and Chanel had come up to stay for the weekend. And in the midst of all the preparations, which included Tareq and I organising the payload of a pick-up truck I had acquired being filled with ice for the booze, a message popped up on my phone from my previous girlfriend. I replied to it.

'Are you seriously messaging your ex?' Chanel asked me.

'Yes, I am.'

'What does that mean?'

'I don't want to lie to you. There are some feelings still there.'

That's what I said.

'Well, I'm not sticking around for that,' she said. She went upstairs, packed her bag, made it clear to me she never wanted to see me again and left.

It wasn't a terrific party that night, if I'm honest. It could have been salvageable if Chanel had dumped me, been unfaithful to me, come at me with a chainsaw, because in all those scenarios there would have been heartbreak but a clear conscience. If one of those things had happened, I'd have felt relief to be free of her and I would have partied all night to get over her and woken up to a brave new day.

But there was no getting over this or away from it.

When you realise you are so spoiled that your desire not to miss out on a good time means you keep your options open, open enough to destroy the best thing you've ever had – well, you can drink and party all weekend, but at some point you are eventually going to have to wake up to the fact that you are still that wanker.

A month later I asked her if she'd meet me in London. I wanted to apologise. I'd meet any place and time that suited her. Please.

She agreed. 'But it's just to say goodbye, Alex.'

At the time, she had me saved in her phone contacts as ABSOLUTELY DO NOT MESSAGE THIS PERSON.

Chanel's friends at work had been very supportive of her when we split up. *God what an arsehole/dick/loser/bastard.*

Standard stuff. All fair. They were just doing their job.

When she told them she was meeting me for a final time, one of her colleagues said something interesting: 'Everything you want to say to him, everything he needs to hear, you should say now because it will help the next person.'

'I'm all for that,' Chanel said. 'I'm all for growth.'

She wrote down on a blue Post-it note everything about me that she didn't like. Then she came and met me in Bill's in Soho, near her office.

'Look, I'm just going to lay this to you straight, Alex.'

She went through her list and at times she had to really peer at the Post-it note because she'd written really small to fit it all in.

'I don't like confrontation,' she said, 'but I just want you to know you are a narcissist. You are self-absorbed. I appreciate that you didn't technically cheat on me, but you emotionally cheated because you should have resolved all of those things with your ex before you started with anyone else. You're immature and spoiled and dishonest with yourself. You've never lived with people properly, not with a partner, never had to share. You're an incredible human being, but at the same time your dad washes your bike and your mum washes your clothes. You are like 15 still. You treat relationships like a teenager does.'

It went on. If I could remember the rest I would tell you, but by this point my ability to think was on the ropes. The whole thing was brutal. I would have stood up for myself if there had been a single thing she'd said that wasn't true.

She finally finished and was surprised, I think, when she looked up and saw that I was crying. I was inconsolable, head bowed, tears streaming down my face, sobbing because I knew I had lost her and that I didn't want to be the man she was describing. And that I was.

And where a lesser human might have come across and given me a hug, Chanel said, 'Don't cry. Just do better next time.'

I nodded, and thought to myself, imagine if she *was* someone who liked confrontation.

'I think it's really important to be honest,' she said. 'Because you've hurt me, and you're probably going to hurt someone else unless you realise what this does to people.'

This conversation occurred the same year as my crash in Poland when a chainring slashed my neck open and I can honestly say that I would rather take another slashing from a chainring than another Post-it note from Chanel.

As she left, she stopped and turned. 'We've been seeing each other for three months just about. What are my parents' names?'

I couldn't tell her. And what really pissed me off that day was that as soon as she'd disappeared round the corner, I remembered.

Tracey. Her mum was called Tracey.

And that just made me hate myself more.

In the same year as meeting Chanel and missing out on the Giro, I set up a charity to encourage young people with bleeding disorders to participate in sport. Sky Andrew is a can-do person; a remarkable, brave, original, funny, genius who makes things happen. He and I agreed that we should take the advocacy work of the Miles for Haemophilia campaign up a notch and that a charity was the way forward. We called it Little Bleeders.

I grew up in a time when exclusion for haemophiliacs was the norm. Little Bleeders wants that to be unthinkable, a relic from a bygone age. *Move More, Be More* is the charity's strapline. It applies to everyone, whatever their state of health or level of ambition.

Through the ups and downs in my career, my visibility in the haemophilia community has been constant, because win, lose or DNF, a haemophiliac who sees another haemophiliac competing in the sharp-elbowed environment of the peloton can be life-changing. But it still doesn't come easily to say so publicly; to talk about myself or accept that I might be a role model in any way. Being young and cocky enough to think you'll win hundreds of bike races, drive flash cars, date lots and think the coach who is training you isn't quite good enough is not the same as being confident enough to consider yourself someone who could help change people's lives.

———

The good thing about totally messing up your personal life, and being alone with no appetite to see anyone, is that you do some housekeeping. I do not mean that in any way, shape or form I cleaned or even tidied my house. But my training routine needed a thorough going-over and I lucked out with a chance encounter in Lanzarote with Charline Jones.

We had met in the past, in Delhi, where she won a Silver medal for Scotland in the team sprint at the Commonwealths seven days before I won my Silver. She messaged me out of the blue: 'I hear you're in Lanzarote. I am too and I'd like to sit on your wheel if you're up for some company.'

We rode together and she shook me up. She could see I was down and suffering crippling self-doubt. She was highly critical of my training. I had drifted away from my coaches at Movistar and stagnated.

She texted me that evening with some training ideas: 'Shove these efforts into your ride tomorrow,' the message said.

I did them and they were very hard but felt good. I thanked her and she texted me another training ride to try and that one hurt too, so I asked for more.

Pretty soon she was sending me all my sessions and I was communicating with her daily.

Charline could be pretty harsh and spoke some home truths. But she was also very positive and energetic, good at motivating me, and we made each other laugh. I was an open book to her, always clear about my strengths and weaknesses. I opened up to her on both a professional and personal level. She didn't ask to see my numbers, she asked me how I felt, physically and mentally. As well as having a sports science background and an insanely sporting family (a mum who played hockey for Scotland, a dad who was a triathlete and Ironman, and a brother who played rugby union for his country – as does her husband) she also had a way of applying her immense emotional intelligence to her coaching that put her, I think, head and shoulders above most cycling coaches.

For a year she trained me on a helping-out basis but wouldn't let me pay her, because she didn't yet consider herself a professional coach. I wasn't comfortable with that, but she was very clear. She was finding herself in that role, she told me, and claimed to be getting a lot of self-worth and knowledge from coaching me.

After a year, however, we formalised it. She sent me a list of what she expected from me in terms of effort and what she expected to be paid. It was a resounding yes to everything from me and she was now officially my coach, and she was outstanding. She messaged me every day to get me fiercely engaged in training and urged me to be less distracted by going all over the place to family and haemophilia commitments. She even banned me from going to the British Grand Prix with Dad because it was a training day. I argued with her about that and lost.

Looking back through messages from her – when she would send me a training session and I'd report back how it had felt and what numbers I had produced – what strikes me is that as well as the technical stuff, she had a way of knowing me better than myself and prompting me to do better in every detail of my life.

Ffs Dowsett you can do more than that.

You've got too much other stuff going on, Alex – you have to focus more and rest more.

No, don't go for a walk to relax this afternoon, go to the cinema so you are sitting down and not thinking.

Your training this month has been fucking quality and the belief a good coach can give you goes a long way – well done.

That belief helped me to my best-ever performance at Milan–San Remo. I'm not a one-day Classics racer, but I love that race and finishing in the front group in 2017 was a lovely feeling. I'm like just about every other pro cyclist in campaigning for shorter races, but they should never change Milan–San Remo, even though it is, at just shy of 300km, the longest race on the calendar. It is one of the most dramatic and exciting of all races and I love the fact that anyone – a climber, sprinter or rouleur – can win.

Cavendish won it by a distance of two centimetres in an amazing sprint duel with Heinrich Haussler. 'When you win sprints, you prove you're a great sprinter,' he said afterwards. 'When you win a great one-day race, you've proved you're a great rider.'

Nibali won it in 2018 with an incredibly daring, unhinged descent into San Remo straight after an astonishing attack on the Poggio. Nibali is a pure climber. Cav a pure sprinter. Cancellara is a pure Classics rouleur and he's won it. That's what makes it a special race and I hope they never ever change it.

Charline also had a firm belief in the profound effect on one's training of being happy. I had learned this before, when I went to Livestrong from the Academy and fell back in love with the sport. One of my texts from Charline contained this line in relation to how her own training had improved since she met Lee, her husband.

If you're happy at home you're happy on the bike. It's all about love.

———

Two months after Post-it-gate, I messaged Chanel, just to say hello and that I hoped she was okay and didn't mind me doing so. She replied and we exchanged a couple more messages. The next day, I texted her: *I just need to know, are you completely done with this, because I've got some things I want to say?*

Then I waited. And I became nervous, more tense than I can ever remember feeling about a race. As the hours and days passed without a reply, it dawned on me that every day since ruining this relationship I had been thinking about it. About her.

Then she replied. *Okay, yes, if you want to come and have a chat, then fine.*

We met in Soho Square. It was a lovely, warm afternoon and the square was packed with people who had finished work for the day and had cans of beer and plastic containers of picnic food from the supermarket.

What unnerved me – shocked me, in fact – was that as soon as I saw her, I got upset again, visibly upset, so it immediately just seemed like a direct continuation of the last meeting, like I'd been sobbing for the past two months. I had no control over this at all, and I wasn't actually crying but I was trembling and struggling to speak, permanently on the brink of tears.

I didn't understand what the hell was going on.

As the young professionals of Soho laughed and chatted and drank on the grass, we sat near the entrance to the square oblivious to them. She said things to me that I hadn't dared hope to hear: that she knew I wasn't a bad person, that she felt I had made some bad choices, and she believed I had been shaped by the world I was living in. Chanel had a theory that cyclists were stuck at the emotional age they went pro. Cyclists don't generally go to uni or college, get their first jobs, find flat shares, go travelling with friends. They don't learn to function as adults in the world like the rest of us do. Instead, they enter adulthood surrounded by yes-men who do just about everything for them.

I'd love to argue with her, but . . .

I spent most of that afternoon apologising, but I also told her that I was ready for something different now, that I knew I had made a big mistake, and was there any chance that she'd be willing to think about giving this another try?

I don't think either of us expected the conversation to last so long that day or to cover the ground it did. She said she knew I was genuine. She said that she knew I was very close with my family and that cycling was my entire life.

'But only for a while,' I said. 'My career has an expiry date. And I can change.'

'I've got my whole life to explore my career,' she said. 'You've only got these few years.'

It was an incredibly generous thing of her to say.

She asked me, 'If we go ahead with this, what does that look like and how is that going to work? I've got my own life to live as well.'

I couldn't believe that she was even discussing the possibility.

'I would be so different,' I told her.

'I'm all or nothing, Alex. You're either in this properly or you're not. That's the terms.'

'Yes,' I said.

Then she said this: 'I think the worst thing you can do is live with regret. Why don't we give it another shot and see what happens?'

That summer rocked. We had an incredible time and, I promise you, I was completely different. And I wrote to her when we were apart, dozens of handwritten cards with long, long letters inside. I know that she has kept them all in a box, hidden away somewhere.

She took me to New Zealand. She showed me Queenstown, Lake Wānaka, Lake Tekapo. And, on a beautiful warm day she took me down to a beach in Christchurch called Governors Bay. The sand was pristine, the water warm and clear blue. Trees hid the rest of the world from view and swayed rhythmically in the gentlest of breezes.

'And you think this is nicer than Frinton?' I asked.

When we got back to the UK, we moved in together and, as Christmas approached, I discovered something about her that everyone close to her knows too well – her extraordinarily deep, profound, excitable love of Christmas. Her ambition when she grows up is to live in a John Lewis Christmas ad.

'When are we going to get a tree?' she asked, in November.

Enchanted by an adult being *this* into Christmas, I played a straight bat and shrugged. 'Don't mind. Maybe get a little tree nearer the time?'

On 1 December, she went to work and I headed out and got a beautiful tree from a farm in Essex, went into Chelmsford and bought Christmas lights and tonnes of decorations and a reindeer, and had the entire house decorated and the tree and front porch lit up by the time she got home. Her face lit up like a child's.

Like racing bikes, living with the person you love is all about marginal gains. She will tell you that I am untidy and can't cook, but that if she's going for a bike ride or a swim or a run, I will set out her shoes and kit and make sure her watch is charged, and I'll set her bike up and service it and download a map for her route, so everything is ready for her and perfect. We are a team. We're raising a family and earning our living as a team, we're having fun together, trying to make an adventure out of life and love.

And, yes, I am untidy and I am really awful at cooking, unless it's an omelette you're after or a bowl of cereal. She looked at some food I had knocked together for us once and laughed, as she tried to work out what it was.

'Just eat it,' I said. 'Don't try and put a name to it.'

'How did you survive before we met?' she asked.

And we both went quiet, me sheepishly because I knew the answer and her while she worked it out.

'Oh, right, yeah . . .' she said. 'Of course.'

I shrugged and smiled.

'Your mum.'

Yes. In the old days, I would either eat out or go to Mum's. I'm not denying it for a minute. We're a close family, we do stuff for each other, we love hanging out. I grew up with a mum who liked doing stuff for me and my sister, and I have been training, either in a swimming pool or on a bike, at 6 a.m. or 7 a.m. most mornings of my life since I was seven years old, and working my arse off and putting myself out there and taking risks. As a result, and because I am incredibly lucky, I have been massively supported by my mum, who has often done things for me like cooking and cleaning to clear a path for my training and racing.

And, also, I'm a bit lazy about things like that. I would prefer to go and do an hour on the PlayStation after training or competing rather than doing the laundry or preparing a meal. I am unique in that regard; there are no other men or women like that in the world.

I completely fucked up when I first met Chanel and I am seriously lucky that she saw something in us to give me a second chance. That mistake I made was in character at the time and totally on me. Chanel had done nothing wrong and neither had my ex. The character flaws I possessed then were also down to me. They were not down to my mum being overprotective or spoiling me and they were not down to me having a rare disease.

But one of the reasons I was a bit spoiled by my mum is that she and I developed a bond of indescribable depth from when I was 17 months old, because a diagnosis revealed that I needed careful looking after and nurturing and my Mum – wrongly, but understandably – felt responsible, having carried the haemophilia gene.

If you think there is anything I, or anyone else, can say to talk her out of feeling that way, then you don't know mothers of haemophiliacs.

Mum has been looking after me extra closely, extra vigilantly, since her and Dad's life was bulldozed by my diagnosis – because I needed it and it was what she wanted to do. Because she is kind and intelligent, she did it while parenting and loving me and my sister equally. I was vulnerable and needed wrapping up. And the bravest thing she and Dad did in protecting me was give me the chance of a more fulfilled life than if they'd done what they really wanted to do, which was to protect me from the outside world, take me home and shut the door.

So, yeah, we're close. She's the most brilliant mum I can imagine and I was too reliant on her until I did some growing up when I fell in love.

Sue me.

13

HEARTBREAK AND GLORY

The Olympics and the Commonwealths

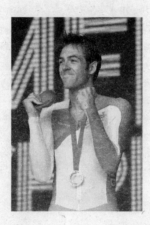

I never made it to the Olympics. And that is always going to hurt. But the variety of ways in which I missed out on three of them is perversely impressive.

As previously mentioned, when I missed out on the first of the three – the one every athlete from these shores was desperate to be a part of, London 2012 – Team GB managed to scrape by without me, with Bradley Wiggins winning Gold and Chris Froome Bronze in the time trial. So, please hear me when I say that in telling you about my unrequited love for the Olympics, I am not suggesting I would have beaten either of them that year. But I will suggest what good bedfellows I think me and the Olympics would have made.

2012 was a momentous year for Team GB cyclists well before the Olympics began, thanks to two rule changes that dramatically changed the sport's landscape.

Firstly, the IOC changed Olympic selection criteria by introducing a new rule for national cycling teams, stating that the time trialist had to come from the road team, thus removing with a tap on the keyboard the specialist time trialist from the Games.

Secondly, the IOC decided to welcome drug cheats back into the Olympics by overturning life bans.

New events are added to the Olympics yearly and very few are taken away. To prevent athlete numbers getting out of hand, the IOC looks for chances to cut back and removing the specialist time trialist from the Olympics was such an opportunity. Decisions like that make a mockery of the Olympics being for the ultimate practitioners of each discipline. It is not the best time trialists at the start line of the Olympic TT, it is people who are there for being the best road or track riders. Sometimes better time trialists are left at home.

Ultimately, my broken elbow in Belgium and the four resulting surgeries killed any chance I had of selection for London, but the change in selection rules would probably have seen me not make the cut when the longlist became the shortlist. David Millar was able to be on that list thanks to the reversal of the British Olympic Association's rule of lifetime bans for drug cheats, after the Court of Arbitration for Sport ruled that such lifetime bans didn't comply with the World Anti-Doping Agency code.

David was a better TT specialist than me at the time. I disagreed with the ruling but not for selfish reasons. Not allowing lifetime bans encouraged cheats like David to consider the gamble. When people cheat, they weigh up the gains against the risks, the risks in this case being twofold: getting caught and the scale of the punishment.

An athlete contemplating never being allowed to race again is a different human being to an athlete knowing that, if they get caught, they'll miss a couple of years and then be back.

It is so obvious that the best way to fight doping in my sport is to have lifetime bans. That's why it was like a Greek tragedy watching Mark Cavendish's 2012 Olympic road race dream get shipwrecked by the peloton's concerted desire to block Team GB and the door being left wide open for a drugs cheat, Alexander Vinokourov, to take Gold. For Vinokourov, who served a two-year ban after testing positive for blood doping during the 2007 Tour de France, cheating at the Tour was worth the risk because he might have got away with it and, when he didn't, he was back on the tour by 2010 and grabbing himself an Olympic Gold in 2012.

In the case of Vinokourov, in my home city, against our greatest ever sprinter, cheating paid off big time. 100%. And it was gut-wrenching to watch. 'This,' Paul Kimmage said at the time, 'is the worst possible result for the race and the sport.'

———

Rio in 2016 was never going to happen for me. The moment my Giro was capsized by the surgery to remove the plate on my collarbone, my chances of impressing the Olympic selectors vanished. And rightly so. When Rod Ellingworth called me to say I couldn't be considered, he was great about it, told me the surgery was just bad luck and bad timing.

It's all about making your mark in the year prior to the Games and when I did exactly that in the lead-up to Tokyo 2020, with a career-best fifth in the World Championships in Harrogate, it not only put me in contention but single-handedly secured GB a second spot in the time trial at the Olympics.

Matt Brammeier, the GB men's coach who also looked after the men's elite brand team at British Cycling, approached Michael Hutchinson three months after the Worlds, in December 2019, and asked him to coach me.

'What's the remit?' Michael asked.

'To get Alex, and Alex's set-up to the start line in Tokyo.'

The appeal of Michael to me and to British Cycling was that he would be across the whole package. He knew me, knew time trialling, knew the whole tech side of it. Michael agreed and I was thrilled.

Michael worked with British Cycling's physiologist, Laurence Birdsey, and the two of them would have a weekly Zoom meeting to look at where I was and what I needed from the balance between recovery and work. They referred to those meetings as *talking about Alex behind his back*. What Michael could do was join up all that with the bike set-up side of things. British Cycling just wanted me as fast as possible for the summer of 2020, whether that was by riding at 20 watts more than I had or getting an aero package that was half a kilometre an hour faster.

'The challenge,' Michael said to me, 'is that you've spent half a decade riding for a team for whom aerodynamics was not so much a mystery as an irrelevance. Ninety per cent of Movistar's knowledge of aerodynamics was in your head.'

His dim view of Movistar's approach to aerodynamics was long established. I had texted him way back in 2013 on the eve of the second time trial in the Giro, having won the first, saying, *What bike should I ride tomorrow? Is this an aero-bike job? There's no one in Movistar who can answer this question for me.*

He replied, *It's not that there's nobody on Movistar who can answer that question. There's no one there who understood the question.*

Matt Brammeier said to Michael, 'Alex is more or less our first selection, because the engineering team is behind you. We've put a lot into this already. He's on the plane to Tokyo unless something weird happens.'

Then something really weird happened.

To the whole world.

The Tokyo Olympics weren't cancelled, they faded away. And that was a problem. When the pandemic hit, the first rumour was that the Games would go ahead but without crowds. Then they were going to remove some of the events. Then they were going to reschedule it to September. What happened instead was a gradual dawning on everyone that the Olympics weren't going to happen in 2020. And throughout those months of uncertainty, in the especially tight lockdown of Andorra, all I could do was obscene amounts of turbo trainer riding on the balcony of our small apartment.

It took a big mental toll on me, training like that, claustrophobically and into a void. There was none of the stimulation of riding with others and cutting through mountain scenery. Instead, it was just grinding away on a static bike. But the damage is not simply in the mind, it's physical too, because there are issues to do with the inertia of a turbo trainer. You're not moving your whole body, 80 kilos at 50km/h. You're spinning a flywheel and what it leaves you with is climber's legs on a time trialist body, and that's no use for anything.

I was better off than most people in lockdown – being paid by my team, living with a view of the mountains with the person I love, and no pressure or responsibility beyond training on a static bike every day and watching what I eat. (On the day the Olympics were finally cancelled, I devoted all my energies to the eating of chocolate.) But having made the move to altitude at long last in 2018, I now found myself in the strictest lockdown anywhere in Europe. In Andorra no road cycling was allowed at all and, when cycling restarted later in 2020, all races were won by riders who had been able to train out on the road.

The key to living at altitude is not doing all your training at altitude. Michael always insisted we did two sessions down the mountain each week, on flat road at a relatively low 500 or 600m (1,640–1,970 ft) where the air was thicker and I could train at time trial speed rather than the constant grinding uphill or coasting downhill of the mountains. When you come down from altitude, you get proper oxygen, can ride at full pressure, with high muscle forces, pedalling hard. The analogy coaches use is that the whole body is like a central heating system. When you go live up a mountain you're doing good things to your boiler and, to some extent, good things to your pipework too, but you're not doing anything for the radiators. To service the radiators, your muscles, you need to come back down the mountain.

Having been in the shape of my life prior to Tokyo 2020, my post-lockdown form was anybody's guess. But I wanted to race and find out how I was, and this led to the only disagreement Michael and I have ever had – my decision to go to the Europeans in France, in August 2020.

'You're not ready for it,' Michael insisted. 'You've had months of terrible lockdown training and no racing. At the minute you're in a very good position to go to the Olympics. You had one and a half feet on the plane. My concern here is that if you race and you're not ready, we're going to go backwards.'

Michael urged me to bank all the credit I had with British Cycling and say I wasn't ready to race yet, rather than underwhelm them in France.

'I'm a bike racer,' I said to him, opting for a bit of what Basil Fawlty called *the bleeding obvious*. 'I've got to race my bike, that's what I do. I can't let a time trial pass me by. There aren't very many of them.'

If you can remember what it felt like to simply take a walk when lockdown was lifted, you'll understand why I wanted to get out and race. Besides, I had contract year coming up and I had to be racing my way to a new deal.

I had made my decision, so Michael supported me and coached me.

On the morning that Chanel and I drove from Andorra to Brittany for the race, a piece of kit being delivered to our apartment didn't turn up until the end of the day, so we ended up driving into the night and arriving at our Ibis Hotel in Plouay in the early hours.

There was something hectic about the whole race. This was partly down to a field of only 28 riders going off at one-minute intervals over a 30-minute course: a quick, busy hour crammed with a hell of a lot of racing. And it was also down to the bottleneck in my career that this race had become. Qualification for the rescheduled Games, coming out of lockdown, team contract renewal – it was all convening at a 30-minute dash.

I was last rider to go. Stefan Küng had caught his minute man, setting a time of 30:18. Michael and I set an ambitious pacing strategy which I kept for the first 10 minutes, but after that I was simply protecting myself and couldn't find the power to attack the inclines. When they didn't time-check me at halfway I knew I was out of it. And the problem was, I was riding well, looking good, the race commentary described it as a great ride. But it was a second-class ride. Fourth best was irrelevant; being 40 seconds and 40 watts off the podium wasn't. I didn't look like an Olympian, just a very decent professional bike rider.

Michael was in the team car. When I finished, he said with typical understatement, 'Well, that wasn't terrific.'

Yeah.

Less than a second off Stefan Küng in 2019 and a minute behind him now. I could see the data arrowing towards the Team GB coaching department. I had worked incredibly hard on the trainer for months and gone backwards by 50 watts. That's what Michael had wanted to keep out of sight until I had some non-altitude training under my belt.

I lay on the bed of our tiny hotel room, with the views out across the car park to a McDonalds, Chanel filming me for my YouTube channel, my team re-signing riders left, right and centre without me, the whole weight and skillset of British Cycling behind me, and I tried desperately not to go down the wormhole of doubt and self-blame. Missing out on the podium by one place – a respectable result in many contexts and to a casual browser of the race history in years to come – felt worse somehow than if I had been way off and able to blame something. But I had raced without problems or injury and revealed my level. By most measures it was not a disaster, but in the specific context of Tokyo it was new information for Team GB – what months on the balcony at 1,800m (5,900ft) had turned me into. Not terrible. Not embarrassing. But Michael was right, it would recalibrate Team GB's view of me. And that *was* a disaster.

And there was an even greater problem waiting for my return: the pro team bike. I was with Israel Start-Up Nation in 2020 and they had the Factor SLiCK. This is the bike that, when Dad and I took it out of the box and first set eyes on it, prompted the two of us to say, in perfect unison, 'What the fuck is that?'

And not in a good way.

Michael described the bike as 'a lump of shit'. This coming from a man who studied Law at Cambridge, has a Masters and a PhD in International Human Rights and is one of the most erudite and nuanced people in professional sport.

He would look through results and send me messages like, *If you'd not been riding that bike, if you'd just been riding an average bike, you'd have come* sixth *not* 15th *here,* eighth *not* 20th, *you'd have won instead of coming* fifth.

'I reckon this bike is making you at least a kilometre an hour slower,' he said.

I began to witness increasing tension between the engineering and coaching departments at British Cycling. The engineers were responsible for developing bikes and skin suits, and working on rider position testing and course modelling. Michael and I worked closely with two or three engineers on all this. The coaching staff, on the other hand, concerned themselves with the hairy piece of meat that sits on the bike and on the results they're getting, what my power numbers were and what Michael reported back to them about my condition.

I was very much a project of the engineers because they had looked at me and decreed that I was controllable and trainable, a serious bike rider who could produce consistent results, and that they could make me faster with a package of technical gains. They had data to be confident I would turn up at 420 watts and further data that confirmed to them that 420 watts would medal at the Olympics. Their calculations included me being out on the World Tour on a disaster of a bike and that not being the case in Tokyo.

But the coaching staff weren't interested in the Factor tractor. All they would say to Michael is, 'He's still not winning races.'

I had been honest with myself early in my career about not having a load more power to find, and that's when I started on my quest for the sort of marginal gains that Brailsford and Team Sky were so right to identify and commit to, way ahead of every other team. I lost out for Tokyo 2021 because my hunger for those marginal gains fell into the engineering culture and, ultimately, they lost any selection arguments to the coaches.

I would have been at Tokyo 2020. It's not unreasonable that for Tokyo 2021 British Cycling's coaches demanded to see better results from me regardless of what bike I was on. I don't find it weird that they took my race results more seriously than my wind tunnel testing. They did not see a reason to try and justify saying to Tao Geoghegan Hart, *You know how you've beaten Alex three times this year? Well, we're putting him in the Olympic time trial and not you.*

It was reasonable, but it was crushing.

———

To the same extent that a cocktail of selection rule changes, injuries and a pandemic played their part in Olympic heartbreak, the opposite forces of good luck and unsuspecting joy characterise my Commonwealth Games experience. I have shared with you the ecstasy of Gold in Glasgow, but just as important to me and my fledgling career at the time was my Silver at the Commonwealth Games in Delhi, when I was an U23 rider at Livestrong.

I love the Commonwealth Games. That's because I did very well at them. You'll find that with professional athletes; the events we do well at, we consider them important and remember them fondly.

The Olympics and Commonwealths would always be on our TV when I was growing up. I'd watch a lot of swimming, but as a family we'd watch any sportsman or woman representing the country. Jason Queally, Victoria Pendleton, Rob Hayles, Paul Manning, Kelly Holmes, Steve Backley, Beth Tweddle, Dean Macey, Gail Emms. They were all in our living room. So, when I got selected for the Commonwealths at the age of 22, it was a very nice moment.

The Delhi Games were on the way back from the Worlds in Melbourne and Geelong. I had gone into the U23 Worlds as one of the favourites, having won the U23 European TT championships. My Livestrong teammate, Taylor Phinney, was outright favourite and he won it.

Representing England was motivation enough for me as I landed in India, but I was also out to prove a point after the Worlds where, at the halfway mark, I had been two seconds ahead of Taylor when I clipped a pedal on a corner. It's not that I would have beaten him. I wouldn't have; he was much stronger than me and I had done a rip around the first lap and was probably going to struggle on the second. But I would, I think, have medalled.

When I clipped my pedal, a tyre came off when the wheel landed. That shouldn't happen. One of Team GB's many, many protocols is that when an alien bike comes in, like my Trek Livestrong team bike, they strip it, re-cable it and put new tyres on it, to make sure that it is up to their standards. My bike was the new all-singing, all-dancing Trek that I'd got after my bike went under the articulated lorry. The Team GB mechanic took it apart and then struggled to put it back together again, and forgot to glue the tyres. That was a mistake, but it was one that only came into play because of a much bigger mistake, me clipping a pedal.

So, no one to blame, but a point to prove. And what better chance than in a men's elite race, not U23, at the Commies? India was fascinating and so was my first experience of a multi-sport games. After the cycling bubble, suddenly I was in a food hall with high jumpers, boxers, swimmers. It was a fun environment. I'd eat with other cyclists and we'd play a game where we looked at people and guessed what sport they did. They came in all shapes and sizes. Presumably, some of them were looking at us and wondering what sport

194

those skinny, emaciated-looking men and women were capable of – or perhaps it was obvious.

There was a boulevard in front of the apartment blocks where we stayed. We'd stroll around there, talk to other athletes. I'd often have a chat out there with Michael Hutchinson, who was representing Northern Ireland in the TT, and then at 6 p.m. we'd all run for cover when a big truck came round fumigating for mosquitoes. David Millar was there. He'd just finished second to Cancellara at the Worlds and seemed untouchable, but I looked at the rest of the field and told myself I could make the leap from U23 to men's here and finish top 10.

The course was flat and featureless, some riders' absolute worst nightmare, because it demanded that you get yourself in the hurt zone and just stay in it, with no let-up. I was used to this sort of terrain. It didn't make me blink. You can take the boy out of Essex, but why would you take Essex out of the boy?

I was off sixth from last. I didn't have any idea of timings, but as I caught Rohan Dennis right at the end – a fact he still denies despite the footage on YouTube – I knew I was doing okay. When I finished I heard a few shouts of 'Fantastic ride, Alex' and the like. Then someone from Team England told me I was fastest. I had five people to wait for. Millar came in 55 seconds quicker, so I knew there was nothing I could have done about that. That is a sound beating. But no one else was faster. I had finished second and, as well as beating Michael Hutchinson, Chris Froome and Rohan Dennis, I'd also beaten Luke Durbridge, who had come second to Taylor at the Worlds. That was the confirmation I was after, in my own head and absolutely nowhere else, that I had been U23 Worlds' podium potential, unglued tyres notwithstanding.

In the days that followed, with a Silver medal in the bag, I realised the Commonwealth Games were bigger than I had perhaps thought and that the Dowsetts weren't alone as a family in having loved them. It wasn't really the response from the cycling world, where winning the Tour de Wallonie is going to do more for your team's UCI standing and more for your own contract talks than the Commies, it was the response from the public to my Silver medal.

You get in a cab in London and are asked what you do.

'I'm a cyclist.'

Then you get either 'Oh, you're a bloody nightmare on the roads' or 'Have you done the Tour de France?'

There's no point replying, 'No, but there's an equivalent race in Spain and Italy, and I've actually done the Italian one and won a stage.'

Because that gets: 'So you haven't done the Tour de France?'

When I reached the point when I could say: 'Yeah, I have done the Tour de France,' it meant something.

Often, you get: 'What have you won then?'

'Oh, Bayern-Rundfahrt, Tour of Poland, the Giro, Tour de Romandie.'

'Eh?'

But try 'Gold and Silver medals at the Commonwealth Games,' and you get 'Brilliant.'

Lastly, it's either 'Are you on drugs?' or 'Can I get a picture?'

Winning and medals matter so much. Silver in Delhi felt just like seeing my name at the top of the leader board as a 14-year-old at the George Herbert Stancer Memorial – which is to say, it felt bloody lovely.

I accept that one of the reasons the Commonwealths mean a lot to me is that big hole in my CV that is the Olympics. But being at a Games for your country is a great feeling, thrilling and humbling, and having a Gold medal placed around your neck is as good as these feelings get. The opposite to that feeling is sitting at home watching an event you've not been selected for. I tend not to do it, but I watched the opening ceremony of London 2012 especially for the segment devoted to the NHS, the institution that had diagnosed me, mended me, cared for me and given me my sporting life. Watching it filled me with belief that it was going to be a great Games for us as a nation and for British cycling. Bradley Wiggins, Ed Clancy, Geraint Thomas, Steven Burke, Peter Kennaugh, Victoria Pendleton, Laura Trott, Dani King, Joanna Rowsell, Chris Hoy, Jason Kenny and Philip Hindes all made sure that was the case. Watching them and that tribute to the NHS made me realise how much I love my country.

The NHS is the safety net for the one in 20 people who live with a rare disease in the UK. It's a safety net that does not exist in many parts of the world. It caught me. That is why I would have loved to have been the first haemophiliac

Olympian. But wanting to be there does not earn you a place. I believe I was good enough to have medalled at the Olympics. But that doesn't mean I deserved to go. I was never good enough or fit enough to be selected when it mattered.

I have to swallow my disappointment, let go of any sense of injustice, because such feelings are rarely warranted when you look at them up close, but I also have to be honest with you and say, I would have loved to represent you all, and I would have pushed myself into any dimension of pain required to do for my country and for haemophiliacs what I did for them at the Commonwealth Games – and I am never going to belittle the achievements of every Olympic cyclist selected ahead of me by pretending it doesn't hurt.

Birmingham hosted the Commonwealths in the final year of my World Tour career, 2022, and I was given a small, privileged peek at the quintessential, behind-the-scenes Britishness of the way we organise a Games. I was asked to take part in the Queen's Baton Relay. As a small group of baton carriers gathered in a cricket pavilion in Essex, prior to our leg of the event, tea and cake was handed round and an organiser suggested we fill the time by going round the room and telling everyone why we had been nominated to be there.

There was a Filipino lady who had raised a huge amount of money for charities in the Philippines, and a girl who had handed out sunflowers to people during COVID (presumably with a stick 2m long). There was also an elderly gentleman who every time someone new walked in would get up and formally introduce himself and shake their hand enthusiastically.

'I'm Terrence. It's very exciting.'

Terrence asked lots of questions.

'Does anyone know what hand we should hold the baton in?'

'Should it be one hand or two?'

'Are we meant to run or is it a walk? I can't run really but I can try.'

It was a very nice room to be in and very British – the lack of elitism and egos, the modesty of it all and the properness, and of course the tea and cake. It got to my turn.

'Hi, I'm Alex and I've won Gold and Silver medals at the Commonwealth Games as a professional cyclist.'

The room went quiet. People stared at me. Possibly they were thinking, 'You? Really?'

Then someone said, 'That's the most Commonwealth Games-y reason for being here that we've heard.'

Everyone laughed. It was an incredibly sweet, funny moment. And fittingly, it was topped when another man said, 'Are you competing this year?'

'No. I didn't get selected.' I smiled, but failed to convince.

The room fell quiet again for a moment. And Terrence touched my arm. 'Never mind,' he said, softly. 'Worse things happen at sea.'

14

MAYHEM

Katusha–Alpecin, 2018–2019

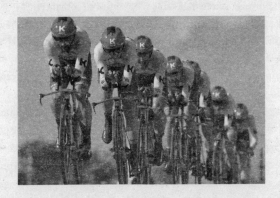

After five years with Movistar, I signed for Katusha–Alpecin for the 2018 season. I was there to win time trials, but my day job would be as team captain in the leadout train for Marcel Kittel, one of the greatest and most exciting sprinting talents in the world.

At the start of my pro career, I had learned how to protect Mark Cavendish for Team Sky. Now, as an experienced though still relatively young pro tour rider, I would be one of the senior domestiques setting Kittel up for Grand Tour wins. Happily, I would remain with Canyon who, in my opinion at the time, made the best bike in the world and with whom, after five years together at Movistar, I had a great personal relationship.

I had changed manager. Sky Andrew, who was never really a cycling man, remained a friend and an inspirational advisor for my work with haemophilia campaigns, but Gary McQuaid came in to manage my career in the saddle. He brought Katusha to the table with an improved one-year deal. The team said everything I wanted to hear: main leadout and TTs, good kit a promise. My gut feeling was that they rated me and I had landed on my feet. I was a lucky lad — and a different rider to the Stage 8 Giro winner of half a decade earlier who presumed he'd be world champion one day.

It was a very international team, with riders from the States, Colombia, South Africa, Australia, Denmark, Belgium, Holland, Switzerland, Germany, Austria, Russia, Croatia, Slovenia, Italy and Portugal. I integrated into the group easily. Everyone got on really well. It was a fun place to be and reminded me of Livestrong in that way.

But we struggled to get results. The problem was Marcel Kittel. He had come from Quick-Step, winning five stages of the Tour de France, and suddenly he couldn't win even the smallest of races. Physically he was more capable than anyone and some of the things he could do, I had not seen anyone else do. But when his head went, anyone could drop him. I've never envied sprinters and the pressure they are under. For all pro cyclists, torment is part of the job. The ability to go through pain and mental anguish is a badge of honour for most elite athletes, because it has been identified as an important attribute you possess early in your rise. It means that a lot of us do not develop the tools for recognising and dealing with anxiety and depression, because what defines us is our ability to push through and ignore what we are feeling and experiencing, and get rewarded for it when we cross the line.

I spent two years at Katusha, from 2018 to 2019, and during just that short period of time Mark Cavendish was diagnosed with depression; Taylor Phinney talked openly about spending hours alone in his room crying in his early career; Victoria Pendleton revealed she had once stockpiled enough drugs to kill herself; and, in March 2019, Kelly Catlin, three-time world champion track cyclist, took her own life.

I have always had my family or Chanel to help keep me from my demons, along with a sense of humour that finds certain behaviours by people and teams in cycling ridiculous and laughable, rather than depressing. And while some individuals and situations have got to me, nearly capsized me emotionally, and I have places of darkness in the mind I go to, I have always been able to climb out again, partly because there has always been someone in life holding my hand. It helped me that I had mates who weren't cyclists and that I lived in Essex, not Girona like just about every other English-speaking bike rider. I liked professional cycling to be my job, not my life, and I succeeded in keeping it that way most of the time, though not always. That's why it came as a surprise to me to discover that, as well as captaining the leadout for Marcel Kittel, I would find myself having to manage his swinging psychological state on the bike.

I went to the Giro in my first year with Katusha. In 2018 the race started outside Europe for the first time in its history. Something had persuaded the Giro organisers that the tour should begin in Jerusalem. Israel paid a reported $12 million to host the prologue. A new name was circulating in the peloton, that of a larger-than-life estate agent from Canada who had been born into a personal fortune and loved cycling. His name was Sylvan Adams and our paths would cross in dramatic fashion before the decade was out.

The team did well enough in the prologue. I was fifth and my teammate, José Gonçalves, fourth. Tom Dumoulin won it, beating Rohan Dennis by a second. It was a promising start, given that I was in a slow skin suit and a very slow helmet. But it would be the deficiencies with the kit that shaped our Giro, not our efforts to overcome them. Katusha didn't win a single stage. The wheels didn't feel, or sound, good and the whole team had serious brake issues in the rain, apparently due to flex in the callipers.

Despite the enormous concerns of myself and my teammates, that year's Giro did offer me one outstanding highlight – rooming with Tony Martin and watching him train his eyes every morning. He'd get up early and stand in the middle of the bedroom with a toothbrush he had put a piece of Blu Tack® on. He would cover up one eye and with the other eye he'd follow the Blu Tack® 10 times to the right, 10 to the left, then take it all the way around as far as he could see and then come back. Then he'd pin the Blu Tack® on the wall and just stare at it for a very long time. Then, 10 times, he'd shift his head quickly to the right and slowly bring it back, maintaining eye contact with the Blu Tack® throughout. Then he'd do the same with the left eye.

After four mornings of watching this, bemused, from my bed, I said, 'Tony, what are you doing?'

'Well, Alex,' he said. 'I crash a lot.'

'Yes, you do.'

'I work with my osteopath, Hanzi, and we figured that maybe there's a problem with my eyes, so I'm training my eyes.'

'That makes perfect sense.'

'Yes.'

'Is your osteopath really called Hanzi?'

'Yes, Alex.'

Tony was a rider I had spent a decade trying to emulate or beat. He was the most unflappable, matter-of-fact German I ever met, and that's saying something. I loved him and he is a phenomenal rider, but his awareness of what was around him was not the best. We finished one stage on the Giro that year where the hotel was only 1km away, so we all rode back to it. We entered the gates of the hotel and the team bus and other vehicles were clearly parking up to the left. The whole team followed them onto the gravel to park up the bikes, except Tony who didn't realise we'd transitioned from tarmac to gravel, hooked a hard left and wiped out immediately.

The eye exercises really didn't seem to be doing anything.

But his mental toughness was as good as anyone's I've known and he was physically very strong. Tony hated being in the peloton where crashes seemed to seek him out, which is why he did so much work from the front where he felt safe. We did a leadout for Kittel. I was on Tony's wheel. He started his lead 20km out and finished it with 1km to go, which is just mind-blowing. His downfall was his ability to crash and I think he knew it. He's retired now and looks a lot happier for it.

At the BinckBank Tour (it's called the Benelux Tour now) in that first year, I quickly realised we had a problem with Kittel. And it wasn't just me, even the race commentators on the first stage said, 'There's nothing wrong with that leadout; that's one of the strongest leadout trains here.'

I was looking after Kittel all day, checking if he was all right. Throughout that first stage race he was saying, 'Yes, I'm fine. You don't need to ask me.' Well, I did need to ask him because as road captain I asked everyone. It was my job to go around the whole team, a few of whom were complaining about their brakes.

With 15km to go, we were all up the front near the line and when I glanced behind me Kittel was not there. He had been up the front all day, but had suddenly disappeared. I started dropping back to find him, but he was nowhere. Eventually, I found him at the back of the field. It had been soul-destroying to give way to 180 riders because I knew it was going to be hard to get back to the front again.

'Marcel, mate, you alright?'

'Alex, I can't handle this. These brakes don't work. I can't do this.'

'Okay,' I said, and watched him and weighed up the options. He seemed fine physically, but the brakes had freaked him out and he'd gone from 'I'm fine, stop asking me' to 'I can't do this.'

'If you don't want to sprint, that's fine.' I said. 'I'll let Rick [Zabel] know and he can sprint instead of leading you out. That's fine. But before I do, just know that the last 4km are dead straight. You're barely going to need your brakes. It's a very simple finish. Let's consider that.'

He grimaced.

'I'm going to stay here with you,' I said. 'If at any point you want to go to the front and do the sprint, let me know. I'll take you there.'

Marcel shook his head. 'No, can't do it. Rick should do it.'

I stayed with him for the next 8 or 9km and then, with 6km to go, out of nowhere, he says, 'I'm going to sprint.'

And it was extraordinary, the way he weaved through the bunch and the huge amounts of power he produced. It was jaw-dropping. It was also infuriating because he finished second in a photo finish to Fabio Jakobsen and if he had just stayed anywhere near the front with us, he wouldn't just have won, he'd have annihilated the field.

Then, on Stage 3, after a Stage 2 time trial, Marcel had a mechanical, got it fixed, got going again and it was my job to lead him back to the front. Every time I went over 500 watts, he'd say, 'Easy, easy. You go too hard.'

I said, 'I'm not going hard here and you're on my wheel. You can't get to the front of this race without going over 500 watts.'

He couldn't do it, or he wouldn't. I was rooming with him and that evening I said to him, 'Marcel, yesterday's TT you averaged 500 watts for 15 minutes. I have never seen numbers like that.'

'Oh, yes, it's pretty good. It's nice,' he said.

'But today we couldn't go to 500 watts for 20 seconds.'

He wasn't really listening. He had his head in a self-help book.

'Alex, you should read this,' he said. 'It's about the power of the mind. You should really read this, it's enlightening. All about the mind.'

'Yes, that's a maybe from me, Marcel. Generally, my legs are the problem, not my mind. I want them to go faster, but they don't.'

We fell silent. I liked him. It's just that I felt our chances of success were pinned on him and I worried about that.

'Can I ask you a question?' he said.

'Yes, sure, mate.'

'Do you think the team's lost faith in me?'

Oh! He meant a proper question, not some chit-chat about chainrings or football.

'I don't think the team's lost faith in you,' I said. 'We all know what you are, what you're capable of.'

He didn't say anything, kept his head in the book.

'What I find odd,' I said, 'if I may, is that I think we have a good enough leadout train for any sprinter to win from our wheel. What isn't making sense to me is that last year you won five stages of the Tour de France from anywhere, with no leadout train. We don't know what's going wrong.'

Then he shut the conversation down very quickly. 'No, that was Quick-Step. You can't compare. You shouldn't compare.'

He put his book down and left. It was strange; it was worrying. There was an important conversation to be had. He was the best sprinter in the world at that time. The previous year he had outstripped Cavendish and everyone else. This year, he couldn't win a club race, let alone stages of a Grand Tour. What was the difference? That was the conversation. Quick-Step had been unfathomably good, with Julian Alaphilippe securing his first Grand Tour stage win at the Vuelta a

España and seeming to be on another planet at times. I wanted him to tell me what had changed for him, to discuss what the difference was between us and Quick-Step. I needed to get into it so that I could do something to address it. But he refused to go there.

———

It took me a while to realise the effect that Katusha and Kittel were having on me; the slow erosion of confidence and my deep frustration that we were a team of experienced, talented, very fit pro cyclists, and that our views and experiences of the kit were being ignored.

The first signs of Katusha's dismantling of my self-belief had come a couple of months earlier at the National Time Trial Championships. On the one hand, the 2018 Nationals in Northumberland were simply about me losing to the best bike rider in the world at the time, Geraint Thomas. No shame in that.

But, in reality, that race was about a hell of a lot more than coming third.

I had been champion at five of the previous seven National Championships, but in 2018 I was beaten before I even started. Geraint had just won the Dauphiné and was about to win the Tour de France, so he was at his absolute peak, but what I had never done in my life before, not even alongside Taylor Phinney as an U23 rider, was look at another rider in the warm-up and think to myself, *I don't think I can beat him.*

I hadn't expected him to be there and his appearance made me fall apart mentally. For the first two-thirds of that race, I was riding the bike but not aware I was doing it because I was too busy wondering how much time Geraint was beating me by. It was one of the rare occasions my dad tore into me after a race.

There was so much shit going on at Katusha, and I knew I was mentally rattled by the knowledge that neither Kittel nor the kit were working properly. My capitulation to Geraint – not even to Geraint's performance, but to the mere idea of him being there – told me loud and clear, as I entered the second half of my World Tour career, that I wasn't mentally strong enough.

One of the worst things Mark Cavendish ever said to me was that I would be World Time Trial Champion one day. It was a nice thing of him to say, and from him it meant a lot to me, but now it was a marker, a cautionary one, because not only was I not World Time Trial Champion, I had just been undone by the mere sight of a great bike rider turning up.

My life was different now, though, because I had Chanel and instead of going into the familiar wormhole of worry, anger and self-loathing, I narrowed it down to just the worry (an improvement of sorts) and talked the rest through with her.

I understood that I needed to work harder than everyone else because I was not talented enough to just turn up and win races, and I was not in a team equipping their riders with the best tools to be competitive. I needed to go and source all the technical information and savvy myself, and make myself a better rider than the one I had become.

I realised too, that summer, that I was not going to be a superstar of cycling. What was still on the table for me, however, was the chance to be an exceptionally good bike rider and to compete and win races. I had fallen, I think, into the trap of inserting the haemophilia story into my professional one as a fairy-tale ingredient. I only ever did this in my own head. Outwardly, I rarely talked about my disease unless asked and even then never in a performance context, only as part of my advocacy work. But somewhere in my head it had always seemed obvious that the way to sign off a rare disease sporting fairy tale is by becoming world champion or winning Olympic Gold. That's how these dreams work out and Cavendish had said that's how this story will go, so I was waiting for that to happen.

I'm not sure any athlete is as successful as they dream of being. It's because we're never satisfied that we push and push and work and work – and that's what makes us elite, world record holders, Olympians, champions. Chris Froome probably looks at his four Tour de France wins and wishes he'd got a fifth. Maybe Geraint has his own equivalent. He won the Tour de France, but he won it only once. I don't know. Until I won the time trial in my first Grand Tour appearance, all I wanted was to ride in a Grand Tour, but then I wanted to win again. Before I completed a Tour de France, I thought I'd be happy simply to be selected for one.

One of my closest and most trusted friends, John, is the youngest of 15 kids and has worked incredibly hard to become successful. We were having a conversation about self-motivation and pushing yourself, and he mentioned a colleague who owns a small Caribbean island.

I laughed, 'Why is this guy working with you or anyone? Why doesn't he just retire?'

'Alex,' John said, 'You've got five national TT titles. Why are you so hell-bent on getting a sixth?'

It's human nature. Whether it be the number in your bank account or the races you've won, you want more – of course you do! If you are the sort of personality that settled for what you had, you wouldn't be at the top of your game in the first place. That's not how anyone gets to be the best.

I sometimes have to remind myself, when I'm ready to dismantle myself and my career in a torrent of self-criticism, how hard I work and have always worked. I have been training intensely since I was a primary school kid. After Geraint put me back in my box in 2018, I knew I had to really fine-tune every detail that could help me go faster, have everything totally optimised underneath me to be competitive, and push myself all over again. If I did that, I would be happy, whether or not it won me more races. And if that meant being a pain in the arse at Katusha, I didn't care.

My one-year contract came to a close and they offered to re-sign me at a 25% pay cut. I felt worried because it was the first time in my career that I had been devalued and that made me feel that I was on the way out. I was incredibly nervous about saying anything aloud about feeling miserable when I was, in the grand scheme of things, unbelievably lucky and stupidly well paid. I wouldn't be able to look my parents in the eye and be negative about the amount I was being offered, and that was telling.

Chanel and I sat down together and talked it through.

'First things first,' she said, 'it's still a lot of money.'

'It is still a shedload of dosh,' I agreed. 'If I ever moan about being offered this amount of money to ride a bicycle, then shoot me.'

'Okay,' she said. 'I promise I will do that. But now tell me what you're feeling, because you're not in a great place.'

'I am really scared of sounding anything like Ashley Cole, but –'

'Who the fuck is Ashley Cole?'

I looked at her and laughed. 'Never mind. Well, he's a footballer who said he swerved off the road in disgust when he was offered £55K a week, not £60K.'

'I doubt you're like him, Alex.'

'Katusha think less of me and that worries me,' I said to her. 'They think I am a lesser bike rider than the rider they signed, but I know that if Kittel had finished off those leadouts we set him up perfectly for last year, they might be in a bidding war to re-sign me.'

Taking a pay cut taps into lots of fears about going backwards and growing old and redundant. It raises the spectre of being on a downward career spiral at the age of 30. That's a bit of a headfuck. It was also the first major setback I had to go through in front of Chanel and I find things quite hard to let go. I analyse things to the point where they just can't be analysed any more.

Another dimension is that to stay at the top you know you can't afford to miss a trick. Of course you're aware this is a lot of money, but you also know that it is the going rate, it's what your competitors are paid and although it might be spiritually wise and morally correct to think, *I'm being paid to do what I love*, there is a part of you that worries that if you think like that, you lack the killer instinct to be at the top.

Where I would have landed with all this had I been on my own, I'm not sure. But I wasn't on my own. I was with Chanel and she loved me, and believed in me, and she was smart and intuitive and knew how to look at things from a healthy, balanced perspective. I had her, I had my mum, my dad and my sister. I was so lucky with my disease that I often forgot I had it. I was being paid handsomely to race bikes.

For fuck's sake, Alex. Cheer up.

I signed for two years because I needed to feel safe financially when I felt so unsure about the team, our star sprinter and the kit we were sitting on. And because I was in love and beginning to dream about having a family. And because Katusha was the happiest bunch of riders I'd been in since Livestrong.

And because I had no other offers.

To celebrate, I went off to the Worlds in Innsbruck and got torn apart by Rohan Dennis. That was 26 September, 2018, the day that finally ended my resistance to moving abroad to live and train at altitude.

Rohan Dennis is a giant. Losing to Rohan is not a problem. But I lost to him at the Worlds by five and a half minutes and this was the guy I had beaten to Commonwealth Gold in 2014, and whose Hour record I had beaten in 2015. Now, I was five and a half minutes behind him.

How the hell had that happened?

The night I lost to him I was sat outside a restaurant in Innsbruck with Alan Murchison. I was bereft, with my head in my hands, asking all sorts of questions not aimed at anyone about where I had gone wrong. I was almost broken.

'I need to do something different. I need to change what I am doing.'

'Comfort kills vigilance,' Alan said. 'You're too comfortable. You live in a nice house on a nice salary with a Porsche on the driveway.'

I gathered myself together before going back inside. We had the whole junior team there with us and they couldn't see me upset. How we conducted ourselves as pros in front of them mattered. They looked up to us. I told myself I would start thinking about this tomorrow, but later that night I sent Chanel a text.

How did I get so far behind?

Innsbruck has amazing air. Even at the end of summer there's a crisp Alpine clarity to it. I remember tasting it, breathing it in, and realising something was changing. I had a moment, stood outside the hotel the day after the race, almost seeing the cool crispness of the air enter my lungs. I knew I needed to stand exactly where I was for a few moments, not just shrug off this defeat and get back on the bus and then back on the bike and go back to how things were, training and hoping.

Breathe, Alex.

I looked out across the town to the outlines of the mountains muscling in on the horizon. I knew what I had to do.

On the journey home I asked myself if it was even fair to raise the subject of moving abroad with Chanel. But when I got back to the home we had only recently made together, the first thing she said to me was, 'Do we need to change something then? Because clearly what you're doing is not working.'

'I think I need to be at altitude more.'

'Okay, so are you going to be on more altitude camps? Does that mean you're going to be away a lot more?'

'I think we actually need to live there.'

'Oh.'

'Yeah.'

'Are you talking about Girona?'

'Andorra.'

'What's Andorra?'

Not *where's* Andorra? *What's* Andorra? That was the scale of what I was asking her to do for my career – move to a small landlocked country so obscure that even a very well-travelled, highly educated New Zealander didn't know where or even what it was.

'I need to go somewhere for me to train more efficiently, at altitude. Not going off on endless training and altitude camps and being away from you. It would be us, living at altitude.'

She did that thing she does when she's making a decision – looked down, nodded her head as she turned things over – then looked me in the eye and said, 'Cool, let's do it.'

Approximately 30 seconds later, she messaged George Bennett's partner, Caitlin, because they lived in the region and she wanted to see how it was for a partner of a cyclist out there. Caitlin gave her the number of the guy who helped people relocating to Andorra. Chanel was talking to this guy, Doug, within five minutes, and filling sheets of paper with the information and advice he was giving her.

We were on our way.

That off season saw the release of the *Haemophilia 180* report into the future care of haemophiliacs. The report looked at why we were spending hundreds of millions of pounds a year on haemophilia treatment and still lacking physios, counsellors and psychologists to accompany medical treatment, and help those with legacy issues like HIV and Hep C, premature disability and the experience of bullying in school.

Many issues were raised. For example, the fact that haemophilia treatment had, due to cost, been rationed in a way that would never happen with a condition like diabetes – no one advocated giving a little treatment to a diabetic so that immediate effects were treated but so little that multiple organ failure and blindness was guaranteed down the line.

On 27 November, I started the day being interviewed about the report by Chris Evans and Vassos Alexander on Radio 2. I did 12 more radio interviews that day before going on to the Houses of Parliament to take part in the launch. Before Dan Hart and Liz Carroll, CEO of the Haemophilia Society, delivered their speeches, Mum spoke to the audience about her experience. She told them she had seen big improvements in terms of treatment, but that she still saw parents and families experiencing the same fear and uncertainty she did when I was young.

The report led to the formation of the All-Party Parliamentary Group on Haemophilia and Contaminated Blood and to the official enquiry into the UK blood scandal. For the families and friends of the 2,500 people who died from contaminated blood, having their suffering and loss recognised would be an important step, just as it was for the families of those who died at Hillsborough. With enormous pride, I watched Mum address the audience in Parliament, and with hope in my heart that haemophiliacs and their parents will one day soon experience complete care.

I entered my second year with Katusha with a lot of hope, too. Despite concerns and doubts about the kit, I was positive about where my head was at and looking forward to attacking the season with a great group of riders. At the UAE Tour, in February 2019, on a mountaintop stage finish, there was a big slowdown in the peloton and everyone grabbed their brakes. I rode straight into Cav's back wheel and went up over the handlebars, damaging my hand.

I got taped up and returned to the race. It was agony trying to grip anything, but it was pain I was prepared to go through. The trouble was not the pain, but the fact I could not hold the bars. The team doctor ordered me to stop. Without a proper grip on the handlebars, I was likely to cause further damage, either to myself or other riders. Although being able to continue racing – albeit barely and dangerously – was a step up from the month in hospital that a broken bone meant as a young haemophiliac, this innocuous little injury, a minnow in the pantheon of crashes and injuries, meant that I missed the next six weeks of racing.

I returned for the Tour de Romandie, always one of my favourites. I rode well for a sixth place in the prologue, behind Geraint in fifth, and everyone was happy. On the first race stage, I was feeling great over the first climb. Ilnur Zakarin, our GC, shouted, 'Alex, you're flying, man!' A little later, I went for a bottle and as I grabbed it my own team car turned left into me and wiped me out. I was rushed to Neuchâtel Hospital with a concussion, strapped into a spinal board overnight and ruled out for another three or four weeks. As I lay there, I thought to myself, *Our set-up is not enabling us to compete, but at least we know the team car is working fine – well enough to run me over*. Sometimes riding for Katusha was like living in a comic strip.

During that second lay-off, there was a team meeting with SRAM at the Canyon headquarters in Koblenz and it got ugly. SRAM had released a new groupset and given Nils Politt a bike to test, with the new groupset and disc brakes on it. But while SRAM were changing us from rim brakes to disc brakes, Canyon weren't changing the bike. The result was a bike 500g heavier. A great bike had been turned into a poor bike with suboptimal aerodynamics and weight.

They asked for Nils' feedback on the set-up.

'It's terrible,' he said. 'It's slower. I don't know, it just feels like it digs into the road, like it's heavier. It doesn't feel as fast, everything just feels worse.'

It wasn't the response that SRAM or Canyon wanted.

But the real problem in that meeting was what Katusha had not told us – that the team was in financial trouble, and it was SRAM and Canyon who were effectively propping it up with extra financial input. Oblivious to this fact, I put my hand up.

'Why have you done this?' I said. 'Everything in cycling now points to bigger chainrings, bigger sprockets, bigger pulley wheels. You've not just stayed where it is, you've gone the other way.'

'We've made up for the efficiency elsewhere.' This came from Jason, the main SRAM guy.

'Where?'

'Elsewhere.'

All the riders laughed.

'What, it's like some Jedi mind trick?' I asked.

That got a laugh too, but not from anyone at SRAM, obviously.

'Elsewhere?' I asked, again. 'Where is that?'

'Elsewhere within the groupset,' Jason said.

'You do know we're professional cyclists, right?' I said. 'And that we are not only capable of understanding where you make up efficiency, but we have to know. *Elsewhere* is a bit vague for us.'

Jason said to me, 'Sure. Absolutely. We get that. Any other questions?'

Hopefully, he has by now realised his full potential by going into politics.

Equipment played a large part in Katusha's downfall. But if a team is in financial trouble and beholden to their kit sponsors, they lose the bargaining position to demand better equipment. On the team, we felt we were starting every race with one hand tied behind our back, then leading out for a sprinter who could no longer sprint. Marcel Kittel was the other main ingredient in Katusha's demise. A lot of us were quite angry that his failures got blamed on the leadouts.

In our opinion, without wanting to get too technical, we served him well and he fucked it up.

I went to see Alexis Schoeb, Kathusha's president, and said, 'These are solvable problems. You need to get rid of SRAM, buy Shimano, get rid of Zipp, buy fast wheels. Then we'll win more races and the thing that attracts new sponsors is winning bike races.'

I also told him the skin suit was slow. 'You've gone out and found a fast material, but you haven't factored in the seam placement and fit. They're both wrong and costing us gains.'

'Have you tested this?' Alexis said.

'No, but Tony Martin had failed to win a race as world champion since he put that skin suit on.'

213

I know it's easy to tell to a rich person who owns a bike team for a hobby to simply throw more money at it, but if you allow inferior kit on board because you are beholden to the manufacturers, you're screwed.

The Canyon TT bike had a dropdown base bar. I was a big advocate for a high base bar because all the time trials now had climbs in and low is an unnatural position for climbing. We were losing time by having low base bars and I could prove it. In 2018, I asked Katusha to address it by giving everyone a flat base bar in 2019. I sent a document with pictures from the Giro showing riders – especially Roglič – doing so much better with a high position. When we turned up at the preseason camp and all the new 2019 bikes were brought out, they all had dropdown base bars.

'Why?' I asked them. 'Did I not pitch this well enough?'

One of the Katusha mechanics was Roger and he used to be Fabian Cancellara's mechanic. 'Cancellara liked a low base bar,' he said.

And that was the team's position. We would all have a low base bar because Fabian Cancellara, who had nothing whatsoever to do with Katusha and who had retired three years ago – a long time in bike tech design – once liked it.

I decided to pick my battles in future. I had lost that one and there were clearly going to be plenty more. I would take care of myself instead. I messaged Erik Zabel, one of the most understanding and emotionally intelligent people at Canyon. Erik, Rick Zabel's dad, is one of the most wonderful ex-pros there is and he was very involved in Katusha and often came to races to watch Rick.

Erik, I've tried and failed to convince the guys here, but what I'd like is a flat base bar or, if you could make it, I'd like a pointy-uppy base bar.

He messaged back: *Alex, I'll do some digging for you.*

He came back quickly, saying that Canyon had made three prototype pointy-uppy base bars that had never seen the light of day.

May I have all three please, for my training bike, race bike and the spare bike?

He sent them. They looked ugly, but I didn't care. I wanted to be able to go up a hill on a TT bike without having my hands around my feet. The other riders laughed as I put them on and then tried them out and loved them.

In April 2019, Chanel and I bundled our cat and everything that we needed into a hired van and drove to Andorra to an apartment 1,980m above sea level, which would now be our home. It was just 55m² plus terrace. I had my broken thumb from the UAE and was absolutely no help whatsoever.

She hardly mentioned it.

Once we were there, I started to panic about the scale of the sacrifice Chanel was making for me. In time, with a conversation here and there, she'd address those fears by telling me:

'I know you can't change your profession whereas I can be more flexible.'

'I was feeling a bit burnt out with work and commuting and needed a change.'

'Your career has to be the focus point for the next few years, because we know it will come to an end at some point.'

'I am up for treating this as a bit of an adventure.'

'But you are in such shit for smuggling your video gaming chair on to that van and into this apartment.'

The first six months we lived in Andorra, Chanel wasn't in Andorra. We spent three weeks there together when we arrived and then I went away to a hefty racing calendar and Chanel found herself alone in a place where we knew no one. So she went to Turkey with a friend and then to Dubai and then to France and then back to the UK. But in time, we met people out there and Chanel got settled into it and we made good friendships.

That hefty race schedule I mentioned? José Azevedo, Katusha's general manager, called me in. The team coach, Kevin Poulton, was in the room too.

José said to me, 'You're on the list for the Tour de France, but you've hardly raced.'

'That's because your team car ran me over.'

'Yes, true.'

'But I've trained well and I'm in great shape.'

'Yes, but you need to race.'

'Totally agree, José.'

'You're going to do the Dauphiné.'

The Critérium du Dauphiné is the final lead-up race to the Tour de France and one of the hardest weeks there is of the year. I thought this was an excellent choice of pre-Tour race for me.

'Great,' I said. 'And, thank you. I'm really excited about doing the Tour.'

'Then, you're going to go to Zeeland Tour.'

'What?'

'And after that you must do the Nationals,' José said, with a straight face.

'That's too much.'

'You have to race.'

'Yes, but I don't have to kill myself.'

'If you do all this, you go to the Tour.'

'On my knees.'

José put a hand on my shoulder. 'Alex, before you do the Tour de France, you have to do this number of race days in the season.'

I said, 'That's bollocks, that's old-school thinking, cramming them all in.'

'That's what you need to do. If you don't do that, you're not going to go to the Tour de France.'

'Then I have no choice, do I? I have to do it.'

The Dauphiné was brutal, but I got through it. It's a beautiful and dramatic race, but had lost its magic for me now that it signalled the start of a long, punishing preparation for the Tour, when it should have been the entirety of it. And if the 4,000m ascent on the penultimate stage, or the six intermediate climbs on the final stage, neither finished me off nor inspired me to greatness, it might have been because we were all still numbed by the horrific crash Chris Froome had suffered reconning the Stage 4 TT. Chris took one hand off the bars (the pointy-down bars), and was hit by a gust of wind and thrown against a wall, resulting in multiple injuries including a fractured right femur and right elbow, and fractured ribs.

My second Tour de France would not, we now knew, be the setting for Froome to win a record-equalling fifth yellow jersey.

As most riders rested up until the Tour, I flew straight from the Dauphiné to Holland, had two days off where I lay down all the time, in an effort to conserve every precious ounce of energy. I did the Zeeland Tour, which started in a time trial where I came fourth behind three Jumbo-Visma riders. Tony Martin was one of them and I got chatting to him, Jos van Emden and Primož Roglič.

'You going to the Tour?' Tony asked.

'Yes, if I complete Katusha's race schedule. I've done the Dauphiné, now this, then the British Nationals. If I complete all that, I'm having three days off, then going to the Tour.'

All three of them went quiet. Tony Martin was staring at me, the other two were staring at each other, incredulous, and laughed under their breath.

'Are you insane?' they asked.

I just shrugged.

I played a game after that. Any conversation I was in with another pro rider I would tell them my pre-Tour schedule and then see if the word *insane*, *crazy* or *mad* came back at me. One of them always did.

I won the TT at the Nationals, the fifth time in six years I had been crowned National Time Trial Champion. This one was special because it was the beginning of the Dan Bigham era, the first time he and John Archibald and their highly talented and intelligent contemporaries were competitive. They almost beat me and it meant a lot to me to fend them off.

And it also meant a lot because it meant I was off to the Tour de France for only the second time in my career.

Exhausted.

Despite all the good times as a team on the bikes, it was a tour that, in classic Katusha style, would be peppered by team politics and the general sense of bedlam that typified my time with them, with every rest day and most evenings taken up by meetings about whether the team was going to exist by the end of the year.

We started to ask questions. 'Look, I still have a two-year contract. If there's an option to go, can we go?'

They said, 'No, you have to respect your contract.'

We said, 'Will you pay us for the whole contract even if you stop racing?'

'No, we can't.'

'Then we have to look for new teams.'

'You can't. You're under contract.'

Marcel Kittel had no such issues, having mutually agreed with Katusha–Alpecin on a termination of his contract. He had sent the team riders' WhatsApp group a message: *I will be announcing soon that I'm stopping racing, but thanks and goodbye.*

By *soon*, he meant 30 minutes. That's how quickly after his message to us the announcement was made. In it, Marcel said he had *lost all motivation to keep torturing myself on a bike.*

We had mixed feelings as a bunch of riders. Some recognised that he clearly had issues; many felt betrayed that he'd given us no heads-up at all; a few riders believed that Marcel had treated us like shit. What everyone felt very strongly about was that we had all taken salary cuts and now faced a very uncertain future because Marcel's form had been so bad. The team had chucked everything at him. They rented out a beautiful house in Colorado for him to do an altitude training camp. The coach lived with him to get him in the best place physically and mentally. They threw more at Marcel Kittel than I've seen any team throw at any rider, and I include Froome at Israel Start-Up Nation. There was a lot of effort put into that – and all of us got nothing back.

But – and this for me was a huge *but* – I also felt that I had witnessed at first hand Marcel's gradual mental disengagement from the grind and hard work of the sport, and from the pressure of being a sprinter. I thought that he deserved some respect for the fact that he was on £1.2 million a year and could've ridden out the rest of the season, collected £600K, and then knocked it on the head that much richer, but he didn't. He just stopped – and I think that showed the mental toll of being Marcel Kittel. I think that showed that he had no choice but to stop.

I found myself withdrawing from the chattering reaction to Marcel's retirement, thinking of the lonely low points of my own career, of the conversation he started and then abruptly ended with me in our hotel room, which so clearly revealed his self-doubt and hinted at a degree of emotional torment. I wondered if I could have done better for him that evening, listened more, been more aware of what he was really trying to say. Whatever the answer to that, and despite how unhappy and worried I was about the Katusha situation, I found myself feeling pleased for Marcel Kittel, even relieved for him, and wishing him the happiness that he was clearly searching for.

We're all searching. He had simply been honest.

15

LIFE EXPECTANCY

The Tour de France

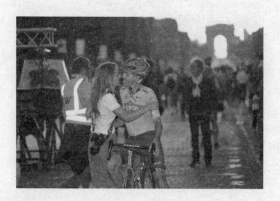

The Alps. 8 June, 2015.

I am riding on a wide road, plenty of space. It is Stage 2 of the alpine Classic, Critérium du Dauphiné. My team, Movistar, will win the race six days later. Everyone in the peloton is in peak shape. The Tour is three weeks away.

A wide road is usually a stress-free road, but 10km ahead is a dramatic bottleneck at the start of a climb. Positioning now is everything and every rider knows it. On my wheel is my teammate, Alejandro Valverde, two-time winner of this race, winner of the Vuelta, four-time stage winner at the Tour de France. He must be perfectly positioned going into the climb. He is growling at me.

'Alex, vamos. We've got to go. Vamos, vamos.'

I glance over my shoulder at him. A leadout rider's job is to keep a cool head in moments like this, knowing when to wait and when to go.

'Wait,' I say.

I watch as everyone ahead of us fights and jockeys for position. One team gets to the front on an effort, sits back and is immediately overtaken by another. The second they win a mini battle, they have a new one on their hands, to get back to the front. I watch this pattern repeat itself kilometre after kilometre. I conserve my energy and Alejandro's. We remain in the bottom half of the peloton, safely away from danger.

Valverde gets nervous. 'Alex . . .'

I glance back again. 'Mate, chill out. I'll get you there.'

We stay where we are.

Everyone else is fighting, fighting, fighting.

We wait.

And then, 1.5km before the climb, I see an ebb in the energy of the front group and I'm out of the saddle.

'ALEJANDRO, LET'S GO!'

I lead him out and we scream up the side of the bunch. The road, two lanes wide plus a hard shoulder, starts to narrow to the size of a small country lane in Essex. The funnel effect is colossal. Alejandro is on my wheel. We don't need to speak, our breathing is in perfect sync, we are tearing past the group. I take him into the bottleneck with me in first, him right behind me in second, and I pull off and ride straight onto the grass to make sure he can get through, and that I don't take anyone else out.

This is the moment Movistar pick me for the Tour de France.

———

Moments like that one in the Dauphiné, those vital minutes where a leadout rider observes and holds his nerve, those situations where you say to the GC contender or sprint specialist on your wheel: 'Wait, wait, trust me, not yet . . .' – on the Tour de France those moments get bulldozed to absolute fuck.

And replaced by, 'Go! Go! Go! Get to the front! No, not in a fucking line, side by side! Go! Fuck! Go!'

On the Tour, you sack off the nuances and fill those moments with brute horsepower simply to stay within sight of the monstrously strong riders kicking the shit out of each other at the front.

Why?

Because the Tour de France is a completely different animal to any other cycle race.

The Giro is more nuanced, in some ways less sane, and on many stages equally draining, but it doesn't hold a candle to the stress of the Tour. It's the relentless strain on your body and spirit that makes the Tour incomparably hard. Even after more than a decade as a professional cyclist, I find that some of the racing at the Tour feels unreal. The breakaway goes faster, then everyone goes fast, proper fast, and for longer. Everyone's dialled to 10 from the moment the flag drops until the finish line. You even have to pee fast.

Because of Team Sky rocking up and riding at the front continually, every team director wants his riders at the front, all the time. And not just a couple of them, the whole team, in a line, at the front. This is what chucks out of the window a leadout rider's principal character trait, which is to be unflappable and scientific about waiting for the right moment.

———

2015 was my first Tour de France.

It was a good year, with my Hour record in Manchester, and winning the TT and the GC at Bayern–Rundfahrt. Movistar were very happy with me. On Stage 4 of the Tour, I crashed, trying to move Valverde up. He was on my wheel, exactly where he was meant to be, and I took him to the front, just as I had at the Dauphiné, but as the gap closed I let him through and was left with nowhere to go but off the edge of the road. It was him or me, and that was an easy professional choice for me to make.

I know my place!

I was critical of myself for that manoeuvre, but in typically, sometimes mystifyingly, laid-back fashion, my bosses at Movistar said that I had done the right thing, was doing my job and had sacrificed myself for Valverde. It was nice of them to say it, but the trick is to get your guy to the front without tipping yourself off the side of a mountain.

Like many before me and since, I have the letters DNF next to my name.

Did not finish.

Movistar won the Team Classification and our stars, Quintana and Valverde, were a great second and third in the overall race for the team. I vowed to return and one day complete the Tour.

It took me four years.

———

Before the 2019 Tour de France I went for a check-up at the Royal London Hospital. I was by then riding for Katusha and one of my teammates asked me what happened at my appointments.

'They're to remind me I've got haemophilia,' I said.

I wouldn't have lasted a week on the World Tour if I had ever sat on a start line thinking about my disease. Even injecting myself with synthetic Factor VIII is as natural to me as pouring cereal and milk into a bowl in the morning. Dan Hart's mission is to get to a point where someone with haemophilia can forget they live with it the majority of the time, and be free of the physical and psychological shackles of the disease.

There's another question I have occasionally been asked by a teammate.

'What's your life expectancy, Alex? Is it less?'

I've always said two things in reply.

Firstly, I consider it the same as a fit and healthy person's. My life expectancy is more affected by cycling than by haemophilia.

Secondly, thank you for asking.

That I consider it the same does not mean that it is the same. While improvements in treatment and care mean that life expectancy for mild haemophiliacs can be near to normal, the official line on people, like me, with severe haemophilia is that you live for ten years less.

But here's how I look at it. My chances of long life have not been reduced by infection with Hepatitis C or HIV the way it was for a tragically vast number of haemophiliacs. Neither are my chances affected by any risk from my synthetic Factor VIII, because there are none. And the way I choose to think and live is that, hopefully, with any luck, the years I put on by being fit and healthy and active will outweigh the years that my rare disease costs me. Because of the sporting life I have sought out, and thanks to the NHS and the pharmaceutical companies who invented synthetic blood-clotting agents, I have the luxury of choosing to quantify my life expectancy not in terms of years on the planet, but in terms of what I expect from myself and want from life.

The time trialist in me wanted to be world champion but is happy with six national titles. The proud Brit in me wanted to go to the Olympics and is grateful for Commonwealth Gold. The little bleeder in me, the toddler begging his parents to stop the doctors puncturing my skin with needles, wanted to complete the most physically and psychologically gruelling cycle race on the planet: the Tour de France.

Some people ask, *What is a reasonable level of risk for someone with a rare disease to take, before it becomes a potentially selfish use of resources?*

Well, if we want to save NHS resources, then rugby, boxing, skiing and kitesurfing all get banned overnight for absolutely everyone. Either that or the people who do them forfeit their right to NHS treatment. Then, other risky sports and activities gradually get added to the list, then the marginally dangerous ones, by which time only wealthy people who can afford private health cover participate. Simultaneously, people who smoke cigarettes or drink alcohol are removed from NHS eligibility, as are all people who break the speed limit. All these people are doing things that are not vital to remaining alive and which raise the potential of them being a drain on the country's resources, either by damaging themselves or damaging others.

But none of those things should happen. And neither should undue restrictions be placed on haemophiliacs. Life expectancy is not just about length of life, but quality too. To those of us privileged to live outside of poverty, life does not mean staying alive. It means living.

———

I arrived at the 2019 Tour exhausted by Katusha's extraordinary pre-Tour schedule and was duly given team orders to go out on a four-hour training ride, when all I wanted to do was sleep. Don't get me wrong, I was excited, but I desperately needed rest.

Having the team time trial early, on Stage 2 in Brussels, was good for us. It meant that as a group of riders we could come together, put aside the strong, pervasive rumours of Katusha's financial troubles, and do something good on the bike. We were all strong time trialists and, with the exception perhaps of José Gonçalves, we were all smart time triallists. That's what the team time trial required, some intelligent riding as well as strength. Marco Haller, Mads Würtz Schmidt, Nils Politt, Rick Zabel, Jens Debusschere and Ilnur Zakarin – we all got along well and gathered to discuss how we could deliver the best time trial possible. Then we went training.

'Mate, you look like shit on that,' I said, with customary eloquence, to Rick Zabel.

'It's so uncomfortable,' Rick said. 'We're at the Tour to do a time trial and this is only the second time I've sat on this bike.'

I watched him. 'Look, it's going to make zero changes to you aerodynamically if you raise your bars four centimetres and widen your elbow pads.'

Our mechanic, Roger, was highly skilled and exceptionally grumpy and did not appreciate doing unnecessary work. Adjusting a TT bike by a couple of inches was his definition of unnecessary. But Rick got the adjustment made that evening and after the Tour time trial said, 'Holy shit, I've never had this much power on my TT bike and felt so comfortable.'

I did the same thing with Marco Haller and Jens Debusschere. They loved the adjustment. Both of them are huge in the shoulders, so in aerodynamics terms we were polishing turds, but it helped them get more power out and they had an abundance of that.

Not being uncomfortable on the bike – as a pro cyclist in the Tour de France: you'd think this would be bread and butter to a team.

People presume that World Tour teams spend 24/7 on the cutting edge, with every base covered, that they apply state-of-the-art tech to everything they touch, think state-of-the-art thoughts in their state-of-the-art heads, develop a state-of-the-art understanding of rider position, physiology and psychology, and eat nutritionally state-of-the-art food.

Well, it's not like that.

The reality is that I bike-fitted half the Movistar team on the eve of the 2015 Tour and I did the same when I was with Katusha–Alpecin, two days before the 2019 Tour started. It's comparable to Andy Lyons sorting my foot position out when I was at Team Sky.

As a group of teammates, we had an intelligent if not state-of-the-art plan for the Brussels Tour time trial and then the coach, Kevin, tried to get involved.

'Right, guys,' he said. 'When you are on the front, you need to be riding at seven watts per kilo.'

Everyone in the room told him to shut the fuck up. That might sound harsh, but when you think your coach is missing the point and you're all being told the team is collapsing financially, that's how things get.

'Seriously, Kevin,' I said, 'please stop telling riders they need to ride at seven watts per kilo, because it's a huge distraction from reality here.'

'We know what we're doing,' Marco Haller said.

'And what is that?' Kevin said.

The room went quiet.

'Riding our bicycles fastly . . .' someone muttered.

Everyone joined in. 'What are we doing?' 'What are those bike things for?' 'Why are we here?' 'We don't know anything.'

'Kevin,' I said, 'We get on front, keep the speed and no one does any longer than they can. Please do not mention power, do not mention watts per kilo, just tell us to keep the speed. We're going to do shorter turns on downhills and longer turns on uphills. Then it works itself out, the stronger guys doing longer turns.'

Kevin is a great coach, but he lacked real-world racing experience, especially in an event as nuanced as the Tour time trial. None of us were denying that when you'd look at the data afterwards, you'd find that every rider had done roughly seven watts per kilo, but that does not make looking at the meter and aiming for it the right way to race. Our way was to chomp along really quick, maintain that and get off the front before slowing it down.

There's a momentum energy that you carry in a team time trial and you feel it on the wheels. If you're having to stop pedalling or you're running up on the guy ahead and having to ease off or go to the side, then you know whoever's on the front is slowing things down. They can't go fast enough to maintain that momentum and need to peel off. Conversely, if you are sat fourth wheel and then suddenly you're needing to produce 500 watts to stick with it, you know the guy on the front is kicking too hard and can't feel it himself. But if he is capable of kicking, that means we've gone too slow beforehand, so it's not necessarily his fault. He is simply delivering it back up to speed in the wrong way.

Everyone on our Tour time trial team knew all these things instinctively. We all got it, except for José Gonçalves, who would get on the front and just park it up and stay there. As the second rider it takes balls to go straight past Gonçalves before he finishes the turn because that makes him look pretty stupid. But it had to be done, many times.

By riding on pace instinct we finished fifth, only six seconds behind Ineos in second place. It was widely remarked that we had punched above our weight and we were all buzzing about it, although I was pissed off that Gonçalves had been the one slowing us down. With Nathan Haas – who I strongly believe should have been at the Tour in his place – we could have got second.

But that Tour time trial did a good job, not in gelling us as a team (we didn't need that), but in reminding us how good a team we already were in terms of working together and liking each other. There was an element of us versus management, given all the uncertainties off the bike, and we had got to a point where we trusted each other more than we had faith in them. It's not an ideal way to embark on the Tour.

Dirk Demol was the head director for the race. I think he had his flaws, same as most people, and the way he conducted himself when things went badly wasn't always pretty, but I liked him. He was well respected because he was the main director in the car for Armstrong, Fabian Cancellara and Alberto Contador. You could argue, though, that with those three riders in the peak of their condition, it's quite easy to be a good director and the real test is taking us to the Tour de France and trying to squeeze a result out of it.

Dirk and Alexis Schoeb informed us that the time trial result had really helped sponsorship negotiations for the following year. We were all quite psyched by the idea that things might get sorted and that we were helping. It had a positive effect, and we settled into the Tour with some good leadouts and decent sprints. I was enjoying it.

Our Tour remained classically Katusha-like, though. Two moments in particular had their fingerprints of catastrophe all over them.

Rick Zabel's dad, Erik, one of the human beings not related to me that I have the most respect for in the world, was driving the course ahead of the Tour and relaying reams of information to the team about what lay ahead. He sent the team express instructions for the riders about one stage finish early on and then one roundabout on Stage 10. But Dirk was not relaying all the information to us.

The stage finish was one that looked like a technical one to us on the bikes and the thing about technical finishes is that once you've got to the front it's relatively easy to stay there, because you can control the pace on the corners. We arrived at the front on this finish, momentarily thought we'd sewn it up, then discovered it wasn't technical at all. The roads were three lanes wide and we looked stupid. We had lit it up to reach the front, blown our doors, and then the leadout started happening and we were screwed.

Erik Zabel was apoplectic. 'I sent you all the information for that finish you needed. What were you doing? Why were you there so early?'

We hadn't received any of the information.

It was the same story with the roundabout. It wasn't complicated but you had to know in advance on which side to take it. Erik had sent that information and Dirk hadn't shared it.

'Go right.'

It's not like being asked to relay the Da Vinci Code, is it?

There were 40km to go and we were all sat in the top 50, well positioned, out of trouble, ready to move up. We hit the roundabout and some teams had been told to go right, most of those who hadn't went left, and that included us. We came out of that roundabout placed 100th to 120th, the split happened straight after that and we never saw the front again.

I can describe the scenery at the Tour de France to you if you want – straight off the bat, the start of that Stage 10 with the roundabout was a place called Saint-Flour in the Auvergne and it is a stunningly photogenic ramparted citadel surrounded by rolling hills and a winding river – but there's a thousand YouTube videos showing you exactly how beautiful it is; how massive the crowds can be, how fervent and even borderline out of control; that the mountains are awesome and some of the villages and towns stunningly picturesque – you can get that from anywhere and anyone. I'd rather tell you that Erik Zabel, one of the all-time greats, was sending easy to understand instructions to Katusha using words of few syllables – for example, 'go right at roundabout' – an instruction I would have even understood in Spanish, and Katusha did not have their shit together enough to pass that information on to the guys riding the bikey things.

You don't need me to set the scene. We know the Tour is an incredible visual spectacle. What you need to know is that after a miscommunication screwed up a stage for us (pick a stage, any stage) Dirk wouldn't talk to us for the rest of the day, which was ironic given that if he'd talked to us about what Erik had told him, the disaster wouldn't have occurred. Dirk was hilarious when he sulked, which was often. He wouldn't say a word down the radio, but he would press the speak button so that you knew he wasn't talking to you. And if you went back for a bottle, he wouldn't look at you. He'd hold the bottle out to you and look the other way, pouting.

Roundabout-gate led to a massively heated team meeting, with Erik wanting answers and a mute Dirk looking like he had a bad smell under his nose. Katusha were clearly shitting themselves about sponsorship stuff, so that might have been it. There were a number of angry meetings and after them the riders would sit together and talk about the fact that we didn't have teams for next year. The racing became therapy, which sometimes produced results. On Stage 11, to Toulouse, we got the leadout spot on. We set Jens up brilliantly and he did the business, coming fifth behind the frighteningly good Caleb Ewan, in one of his three stage wins, Dylan Groenewegen, Elia Viviani and Peter Sagan.

We were pleased with a good day's work, but José Azevedo came in to the room that evening as we ate dinner and said, 'I'm disappointed that you're celebrating this result because we shouldn't be celebrating fifth place.'

Marco Haller stood up. 'José, what are you expecting? Every rider in front of Jens today, and there were only four, is paid over a million and they're all sitting on way better kit. This is a win for us because we're a leadout team with no sprinter. Kittel has gone and none of us know what the hell happened there. This is the best it's going to get. That's what you brought to this Tour de France.'

Jose didn't say much. He tended to back down from confrontation and Marco didn't mind it at all.

I was dog-tired for the second half of the Tour and struggling to make it through each day. What helped was that as a group of riders we had a laugh and talked everything through, and my determination to make it to Paris kept me going. Even better, Chanel was working on the Tour, so I would see her at start and finish lines. Although saying goodbye to her and returning to the team every evening was a wrench, it was wonderful to be able to grab precious time with her each day.

She liked to remind me that she got selected for the Tour before me, by ASO who own the Tour de France. They employed her to interview English and German riders for their channels in those two countries. By her own admission, her non-existent understanding of the German language was matched by her knowledge of cycling at the time. Chanel, Marco and I created a hit list of all the riders that she needed to interview and whether we thought they'd be nice to interview (the vast majority) or act like dickwads. Everyone exceeded our expectations.

She interviewed Ollie Naesen of AG2R La Mondiale, misreading the Belgium flag on his sleeve as the German flag because he had his arm up. When she instructed him to answer the questions in German, he had the audacity to claim he didn't speak German and was from Belgium, which she decided was him playing a practical joke on her, possibly egged on by Marco or myself. That led to a stalemate, with her refusing to believe he wasn't German and unable to speak German for her. It was all sorts of awkward; she genuinely believed he spoke German, and he thought she was – well, I don't know what he thought. When Ollie had ridden off, a journalist who had watched the whole encounter sidled up to Chanel and whispered, 'You know that's the Belgian flag on his kit, right? He really is from Belgium.'

Within days, a big portion of the peloton were greeting Ollie every day with *Guten Tag*.

———

By Stage 19, I was on my hands and knees. And I was an uncle. Three days earlier, my sister, Lois, had become a mum. I had rarely felt more homesick, but mother and baby were in great shape and that was all that mattered. I had been struggling to eat for a few days and was feeling exhausted when I climbed on the bike at the start of each day. I had slept terribly the night before in Saint-Jean-de-Maurienne and didn't feel well.

I said to Chanel before the race, 'I'm in serious trouble today.'

'You'll get through it. I know you will.'

The crazy number of race days in my run up to the Tour had caught up on me and now they were biting me in the arse. My race had become about hanging on for grim life and getting to Paris. I had to do that. I needed to stand up at Little Bleeders events as a rider who had finished the Tour de France. You don't inspire people who are embarking on their own difficult journey by not completing your own.

Stage 19 was a short, punishing 89km to Tignes. It was steep leading up to the start line and even there it was fast. Four of us from Katusha were dropped in the neutralised section, that's how bad our start was. Two got back, but Jens Debusschere and I didn't. I needed five minutes at 480 to 500 watts to remain in the bunch, an easy-ish task normally, but I simply did not have that left in me.

Jens and I had our team car behind us and the broom wagon behind them. It's a truly awful place to be and it was a new experience for me. As Jens and I rode alone, what went through my mind was the positive (*we are so close to Paris*), the negative (*tomorrow is a continuous uphill horror day and even if I make it through today, I can't make it through tomorrow*), and the positive again *I've got Jens with me and Jens has me with him*).

The positives outweighed the negatives, or outnumbered them, at least.

'Jens, what do we do?'

'We finish. We're going to fucking finish this stage. If we're in, we're in. If we're out, we're out. But we are going to finish.'

That was the only way to go, finish and then find out if you're within the time cut and still in the Tour. The idea of missing the cut after 19 of the 21 stages was almost enough to make me physically sick.

'Okay,' I said. 'I've got nothing else on today.'

For any other race, you take a view: *pull out now and start working towards the next Grand Tour or classic*. But not the Tour. You give everything to stay in it if you possibly can. Different rules apply to your thinking. You don't weigh up the pros and cons of continuing, you cling on to your place and refuse to let go of it.

All this time, the guys in the broom wagon were calling to us, 'Just get in. You're done. You're too far behind. You're not going to make it.' The broom wagon is the vehicle that rides at the very back of a cycling road race, just beyond the end of the internet and the place where the sun don't shine. It 'sweeps up' stragglers who are unable to make it to the finish within the time permitted.

'Come on guys, get in.'

'No thanks. Lovely offer, but do fuck off.'

Jens and I turned away from them and grunted manfully to signal our resolve, and got hit by a hailstorm.

In July.

We rode on. Jens looked after me. I looked after Jens. We received updates on the time limit. We were inside the cut, but it was horribly tight and there were quite a few climbs ahead. Fortunately, Jens and I were very equal on the climbs that day – both diabolically bad. It kept us together. But the penultimate climb was a big one that went up to altitude, and that is where Jens and I started to differ, because I lived at 2,000m and Jens lived in Belgium, at possibly 3m, depending on how sloped his driveway was.

Jens couldn't keep up. I kept hanging back but eventually he said, 'Alex, you gotta go.'

'No, Jens.' It was like a scene from *The Last of the Mohicans*. 'I'm not leaving you today.'

'No, Alex. Save yourself. You might make the time cut. You have to go.'

(Okay, he didn't say *save yourself*, but the rest is bang on.)

'No, Jens.'

'Fuck off, Alex! Go!'

Jens eased to the side of the slope, let the team car through so it stayed behind me, and then went back to the middle and blocked the broom sweeper. His thinking was that I could take a few sticky bottles (when someone in your team car hands you a bottle and both he and you hold on to it for a few seconds, to give the rider a quick 'lift'), but I'm not really a sticky bottle sort of person and, anyway, as I went up round the corner, I decided I couldn't leave him. We were, by this stage, practically married.

I eased off and waited for him and we continued the rest of the climb together. We were halfway up the Col de l'Iseran when a message came down the radio. The race had been stopped. The hailstorm had caused a mudslide up ahead, near the start of the final climb to Tignes. The summit of the Col de l'Iseran would be the official finish line – and we were nearly there.

The team car came alongside: 'Get to the top and you've done the race.'

I started laughing so hard on the bike that it hurt. But, by then, every single part of me hurt. We were met by a total shambles at the top of the hill. There was no finish line, just a collection of cars down at the bottom. I hopped in the back of one with my Katusha teammates.

'Everyone finishes, there is no time cut,' Marco said.

Jens and I lived to fight another day. And I grinned like a madman and tried to ignore the fact that my body was utterly, totally empty.

The next day, the penultimate stage, was a short punchy final mountain race with a horrific and savage 33km continuous climb to the finish at 2,300m in Val Thorens. Of the 3,366km we covered on the Tour, this particular climb, averaging 5.5%, sometimes hitting 9%, was the 33km of the Tour de France that confirmed for me that pro cyclists are immensely messed up in the head.

I had always known that you've got to be pretty different to be in the peloton, but sometimes I don't think I'm different enough. Not that extra-special kind of different, *off the charts*, *oddball*, *uncommon*, *slightly away with the fairies* kind of different. Thomas Löfkvist, a good friend, said to me when I was a neo pro, 'Alex, what you have to learn is, you don't have to be stupid to be a pro bike rider, but sometimes it helps.' On this particular day, it seemed mandatory.

When we started the climb there was a small breakaway and I was thinking, *This is great. We're just going to cruise up here, a nice big grupetto, and everyone's going to be cool and tomorrow I can go on a nice bicycle ride to Paris and feel like a million dollars. It's all beginning to calm down.*

But what ensued was a full blown, lit touchpaper race between 90% of the peloton up this climb, even though only 10 of these guys were fighting to actually win the race. Everyone raced. It was the peloton's version of the playground game of British Bulldog. It was a storm of insane, wriggling, pumping, helmeted psychopaths. Incredibly, a huge bunch of riders recorded their all-time, one-hour, best power on Stage 20 of the Tour de France. Going uphill.

I was incredulous.

How are they not ruined? I thought. *How can they do that? Why are they not absolutely wrecked like I am?*

And the best bit of all? Team AG2R Citroën decided to have an internal race on the climb, notwithstanding any other teams, and the loser was paying for the beers that night. They raced for beers up the final mountain of the Tour. It was batshit crazy. Riders are ridiculous. It was insane. It was great and it had completely distracted me from the pain in my body. I had finished the Tour, just like Chanel had told me I could and I would. I'm independent-minded, sometimes bloody-minded, but to listen to her and know that she sometimes knows me better than I know myself made me not the first rider to cross the finish line at Val Thorens, but the luckiest.

That evening, I was physically and mentally so tired that I felt an enormous peace. And after the intense and, sometimes, seemingly endless demands on your mind and psyche that is the Tour de France, I realised in the worn-out calm of the evening of 27 July, 2019, that two of the best experiences, on a human level, of my professional career had taken place in the past two days of racing: the deep bond of riding with Jens with an unspoken commitment to getting each other over the line, and the pure joy of watching the crazies in the peloton race up one last long climb at the close of the 20th day of hostilities. I felt proud and happy to be a professional bike rider.

Throughout my career, I wasn't in awe of the great riders. I neither worshipped nor feared them, but I don't think I ever stopped being the guy who could not quite believe he was racing among them. That's the thing I can't put my finger on. In the same way that, to me, the Maldon 10 is as important as a stage of the Giro or Milan–San Remo, I was not surprised when I beat the greats like Rohan Dennis or Bradley Wiggins and Geraint Thomas, yet I remained amazed at being in their company.

I am a professional athlete at the elite level of an extraordinary sport, and I've done some winning at that level which makes people curious about how I got there and can do what I do. But, in turn, I myself sometimes look at the racers around me and think, *How on earth do you do that?*

I was enormously happy for Egan Bernal, the young Colombian who would be crowned champion the next day. Watching the highlights that evening of the penultimate stage and the footage of Geraint letting Bernal past and holding his hand as he ushered him across the line was pure class. There's no better way to be crowned than with the congratulations of the outgoing champion, your own teammate, and someone as accomplished as Geraint. It was great to watch.

Everyone on the Tour who knew me considered Katusha expecting me to do 13 stages and two National Championships time trials in the 21 days before the Tour started to be either stupid or spiteful. I think it was neither, just a mistake, one of many they made. I don't think they had a spiteful instinct anywhere in them. I always knew it was wrong, but I was prepared to do it to because I was going to be on this Tour, and finish it, even if it killed me.

Stage 21 to Paris is a procession, followed by a sprint, and it's in the evening, so there's enough time to sober up from the night before. The team buses had driven through the night to Paris. We were driven to an airfield and flown to the outskirts of Paris, from where we were taken to the start area in Rambouillet.

The stage is painfully slow at first, nothing more than a photo opportunity on wheels, champagne glasses in the hands of the jersey wearers. But the forest of Rambouillet is beautiful and shady, and it's a nice way to wake up to the fact that you are on your way to the Champs-Élysées. Coming out of the forest, the whole race began to pick up speed, as if realising that we did still have to cover 130km and a couple of climbs before nightfall.

We arrived in Paris with 60km to go. I was unsure of my bearings. I got the sense of getting closer to central Paris; the buildings became taller, older, the streets more packed. But I had no sense of where in Paris we were and then, suddenly, we switched a left onto the pavement and I realised that we were whipping past the Louvre pyramid and on to the cobbles of the Champs-Élysées for the first of eight laps of the circuit. The peloton was huge and going at 50km/h. Three or four riders made breaks, but were caught. The sun was low, golden, casting long shadows on to the cobbles and backlighting the trees, and it would have been impossible to ignore how beautiful that city is, how classy and timeless the buildings are. Paris is no Chelmsford, but it looked pretty good and didn't disappoint that evening.

I was on Peter Sagan's wheel and he was in the process of winning his seventh green jersey in the space of eight years. His hair was dyed green, his teeth, his eyebrows, everything. And in his treacle-thick, nasal voice he was mimicking the riders who were savouring the moment around him, calling out, 'Oh, wow! Paris is amazing! We did it everyone! Wow!' I eased away from him out of earshot.

You're not spoiling this for me, Peter. I don't give a monkey's how many times you've done this.

The most photogenic moment for the viewers is the most manic for the riders. The gradual rise up to the Arc de Triomphe with the sun setting behind it, although a stunning visual, means you can't see shit. You power on and hope not to hit the wheel in front that you are blinded from seeing. Then you get round the iconic landmark and breathe a sigh of relief at putting the sun behind you. Suddenly you're doing 70km/h down the cobbles and there are chains flying off, handlebars bouncing, bottles flying everywhere, expletives filling the air.

I was in the top 20 with 2km to go, in between Alexander Kristoff and Caleb Ewan, two of the favourites to win the sprint, watching as both of their chains fell off. Caleb calmly kept the pressure on, shifted into the little ring to drag the chain back over, and shifted back, dragged the chain back up onto the big ring and carried on – and won. Such skill amid a scene of carnage. Kristoff couldn't do the same and fell away, with everything he had remaining in this race for undone by the cobbles.

The final sprint kicked in 300m from the line and Caleb nicked his third stage win of the Tour. Filling my every thought and sensation now was the satisfaction of finishing. I am someone who tends to look forward, not back, but for a moment, as the finish line of the Tour de France came into view, I glanced down at the familiar sight of my legs powering on and the ground hurtling past beneath my pedals and in a vivid, heightened moment I imagined the many places I had sped over on my bike, from my ride to school, to the first races, the Maldon 10, the unwelcome climbs in Italy with the Academy, the dead straight highways of Colorado with Livestrong, the velodrome floor in Manchester, the blood pouring from my neck in Poland on to my skin suit. And I had the sensation, for just a fractional moment, of being back in the school library, head bowed and staring at books and wanting desperately to be outside, playing, moving, competing, like the rest of my friends.

I looked up. I was on the Champs-Élysées. There were dozens of cyclists around me and thousands of cheering people. Paris was drenched in a golden light and my heart was almost ready to burst with a simple, childlike joy at having made it through the most challenging bike race in the world, that I grew up with no expectation of ever being able to take part in.

As I rolled across the line, my body shivered.

Erik Zabel was the first person I saw. You know how sometimes, when you're a kid, one of your mates has a mum or dad that you think is great and you really want them to like you? Rick Zabel's dad was the equivalent of that in bike racing. I always loved it when he was with us on the team at Katusha. He is one of the few former pros for whom it doesn't matter what you have and haven't won or what level you're at, he gets it, he understands what you do and how hard you work and, perhaps surprisingly given how successful he was, he hasn't forgotten how tough it is for everyone.

He appeared on the Champs-Élysées out of nowhere and gave me a big hug, kissed me on both cheeks.

'Well done, Alex! Well done!'

There's no other biking professional I would rather have shared that moment with than him.

Very quickly after that, Chanel and I found each other and we had a cuddle. And in that strange way that often characterises the best moments, the biggest achievements, there wasn't much to say, we just put our arms around each other and took it all in, with big, stupid, grins on our faces.

A massive night on the piss ensued. As I raised the first beer to my lips, I stopped and reflected on what had just happened. The Tour demands psychological strength and to find it you have to dig deep. The result is a perverse mixture, where you go on a profoundly personal odyssey while having 12 million roadside spectators so close they can touch you. You have 197 other riders competing against you and all around you and yet, to get through it all, you have to be with the most solitary part of yourself. It is a totally private affair, watched by three billion people on TV.

That first sip of beer tasted better than any before or since. *I am done with this race*, I told myself. *I do not want to come back.*

Because that was disgusting.

16

AN ARM AROUND
MY SHOULDER

The Worlds, 2019

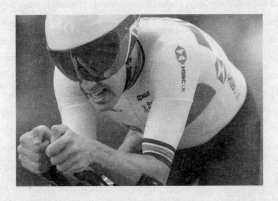

Just when I needed it most, amid all the self-doubt caused by the mess at Katusha, my capitulation to Geraint and falling behind Rohan, I felt an arm around my shoulder.

It came in the form of a call from Tony Purnell at British Cycling, shortly after the Tour de France.

'Alex, our view is we think you've been woefully neglected as a professional cyclist. We're going to chuck everything at you. Your position on the TT looks like crap. You've been let down. We want to turn you into a better time trialist for Tokyo.'

Wow, I thought, someone believes in me again.

Tony Purnell is the global messiah of aerodynamics. He used to run Jaguar's F1 team, then worked for the FIA. Cycling was a hobby for him, yet he became revered within it for his work on strength, conditioning and, predominantly, aero.

British Cycling got to work on me and found that I wasn't as far off as they had thought. My position was unusual in that I had wide elbows and was quite high, but I still tested fast. They found a few small gains in my position on the bike, but the significant gains were found in putting me on different equipment to my Katusha set-up.

A look at my team contract confirmed that when I was working with Team GB I could use whatever kit I chose. The national team took precedence over all else and what mattered to me about that was the freedom to base my set-up with GB for Tokyo on science, not sponsorship.

I told GB I wanted to stick with the Canyon. I believed it was a fast bike, but I also wanted to do so out of respect. I had been with Canyon for seven years and captured the Hour record with them. GB agreed. They believed a Canyon or BMC were the fastest options.

'But,' they said, 'we are going to change your front wheel, front tyre, the rear jockey wheels, the saddle, the helmet, the overshoes, pedals and handlebars from what you have at Katusha.'

'Fine by me,' I said.

During the Tour of Britain, by which time Team GB were deep into their preparation of my bike and set-up for the Worlds three weeks later, José Azevedo, Katusha's General Manager, took me aside in what was an increasingly tense and unhappy atmosphere.

'Hey Alex, World Champs coming up. Are you riding?' He knew full well that I was.

'Yes, I'm doing the TT.'

'Oh, cool, what equipment are you riding?'

'Well, I'm changing just about everything.'

He nodded thoughtfully, then pulled a De Niro grimace, without any of the intimidation factor. 'Oh right, well, we're going to have to ask permission from the sponsors first.'

I felt uneasy but couldn't tell if it was panic or I was simply annoyed at myself for having told him. 'Actually, no, José, we're not going to have to.'

'Well, of course we do.'

'Read my contract. I'm staying with Canyon out of respect, but that's it.'

'Alex, we have to ask the sponsors, out of respect to them.'

'José, out of respect to the sponsors you can tell them what I'm doing, but do not ask because if you ask they will say no and then you've got a bigger problem. While we're on the subject of respect, José, I'm racing for my career at the Worlds, because we've got nothing for next year, have we? I'm literally racing for my future, because no one will tell me if Israel Cycling Academy are taking me on from Katusha.'

'Well, I'm fighting for my career as well.'

'The difference, José, is you can walk away right now and I can't.'

He went quiet, presumably because he knew this difference was a significant one. I was one of 11 riders who had a contract for the following year, which is why I couldn't just walk away and find another team like José could. I was tied firmly to the mast of a sinking ship and he was eyeing up the lifeboats.

'Whatever,' he shrugged. 'You're going to have to talk to Alexis.'

Alexis Schoeb was the boss of the team, the boss of José. He was a Swiss lawyer and running the team seemed to be like a side project for him, which hints at the problematic set-up of professional cycling. But he was a very nice guy to deal with.

He said, 'Alex, you're right. You can do whatever you like. Just please, if you don't mind, try not to put anything on social media about it, not draw attention to it, because we're in a bit of a situation here.'

'Yes, of course,' I said. 'It's not something I would've done in the circumstances anyway.'

It's always good when you get to talk to a grown-up.

The *bit of a situation* was Katusha–Alpecin struggling to pay its riders (I went four months without being paid and found it very stressful), but forcing us to respect our contracts by staying put while management tried to save the team. It was public knowledge that Katusha's way of saving the team would be to sell its World Tour licence to Israel Cycling Academy, who would then become a World Tour team for the first time. The 11 of us had no guarantees that our contracts would be respected, but were bound by a contract that left us watching on as the other World Tour teams filled their spaces for the following year.

Going into the Worlds in Harrogate in late September, I was doing a decent job of putting all of that out of my head until I received a phone call from my manager, Gary McQuaid.

'Katusha have contacted me to say that Israel Cycling Academy have taken over the licence and you are not on their list of riders.'

'Uh, huh . . .'

'They've said you can go elsewhere.'

'Except I can't because it's late September and every World Tour team has been filling their rosters for the past six weeks.'

'Indeed.'

For those six weeks, I had been contractually barred from looking for a new team. And in those six weeks, Sylvan Adams, the billionaire owner of Israel Cycling Academy, had been signing up a load of new riders until there was no longer space for the 11 riders he had told Katusha he would keep.

'Well, obviously now's the point that they need to respect the contract,' I said, 'and pay me for the rest of this year and next, because that's what they've been telling us all year.'

'Absolutely,' Gary said. 'They can't get away with this.'

And with that on my mind, I headed to the Worlds.

Geraint Thomas pulled out of the Worlds TT having failed to retain his title at the Tour de France. John Archibald got drafted in at very short notice. The significance of a home Worlds cannot be overstated and, although it pains me to say it, Yorkshire is the home of cycling in this country. It was a massive occasion and the stakes in Harrogate could not have been higher. Not only were we all racing for places at Tokyo 2020, but if either myself or John finished in the top 10, then it would secure an extra place in the Olympic time trial for Team GB.

I had personal business to attend to as well. I was returning to the scene of a crime. The previous Worlds in Innsbruck had seen me destroyed by Rohan. This time around, I had both the backing of Team GB and the responsibility of being number one, in Geraint's absence.

What I also had was an appreciation greater than ever of being able to roll up to the start line as the National TT Champion. I had won my sixth national title in Norfolk three months earlier and it had meant more to me than the others, because I had had to fight off the frightening, emerging talent of the Huub boys, racing for Ribble Pro Cycling.

It's worth me taking you back to those Nationals in Norfolk to set the scene for what transpired after the Worlds. The Nationals were, as mentioned, the final stage of my dubious pre-Tour schedule. I had enjoyed a run of being National TT champion five times since 2011. Then the Huub boys arrived on the scene. They made a lot of noise. They were very sure of themselves. They described themselves as disruptors. They were very quick on the track and I was a big admirer. The way they did a team pursuit was unlike anything the world had seen. They were a bunch of phenomenally talented, strong, intelligent, scientific riders who didn't care what people thought of them. And the stories emanating from their shared house in Derby suggested they were having a blast.

Dan Bigham reinvented the team pursuit and got national teams scratching their heads and wondering if they were doing things right. They were beginning to make mincemeat of British cycling's best. In 2019, I knew the national title was mine to lose and I was feeling seriously threatened by Dan, John and the rest of their team.

I won it, but beat John Archibald by only a slim six seconds. What was alarming was that John is taller than me, heavier than me and he had put out 35 watts less than me, and I had only scraped past him. If he found five watts, which he surely would, I was in trouble. He was threatening to beat me at my own game of taking on pros with more power and beating them with efficiency.

Dan Bigham then said in an interview, 'John arguably should have won that race.' What transpired is that John had hit a pothole with 1km to go and his chain had come off. I don't know how quickly he got his chain back on, but it could well have been the difference.

But.

Part of the skill of time trialling, and racing a bike in general, is avoiding potholes (and crazed placard-holding spectators and soigneurs swinging food bags and TV crews) while going as fast as you can. The art of time trialling is not going as fast as you can and complaining when you hit something.

I messaged Dan. It was a bit childish of me, but I knew these guys were going to be a problem and they were rattling me.

John arguably should have won the race. What argument is that?

What Dan and his team had discovered was that riding with your head down, not looking where you're going, was a massive aerodynamic gain. The problem with that, however, is that you're not looking where you're going.

Dan replied that his comment was perhaps a bit unfair.

I shouldn't have sent that message, but it had got to me that someone I admired so much, Dan, was being less than gracious about me winning a record-equalling sixth title. The sixth had meant the most precisely because it had been a proper battle with the new generation who had so much knowledge of aerodynamics and who were, I knew, the future.

Yorkshire hosted the Worlds perfectly. The atmosphere was buzzing at the start line and in Harrogate it was phenomenal. Even in some deeper rural stretches, I would pass dense crowds on wooded climbs and they'd spur you on but make me wonder where they had come from.

Rohan had walked out on his team during the Tour de France and was an unknown quantity mentally. Roglič was a favourite and we were wondering what a 19-year-old Remco Evenepoel would do, having by-passed U23s and come straight to the men's elite race from his Worlds' junior title 12 months earlier.

It was a long course: 54km. It started with a deceptively pleasant flat first 15km and after that it was lumpy and challenging, with a couple of minor climbs, but frankly it was the sort of course I had often proved myself highly capable on. We were 58 riders going off at 90-second intervals. I was out bang in the middle of them, just before Filippo Ganna. John Archibald was one of the first away and set an early benchmark of 1:08:16.

Chanel had driven up to Harrogate with Abbie, partner of New Zealand rider Paddy Bevin, and was tense. Mum and Dad were there and the three of them were interviewed by Clare Balding on the media platform above the finish line. Chanel answered the questions, Mum looked off-the-scale tense, setting new standards even by her own on that front, and Dad pretended to be listening while in fact concentrating on the race updates.

I got off to an average start, but I was feeling good. Luke Durbridge was fast, but I came through the second check point 14 seconds faster than him, before Filippo Ganna put the same gap on me. John Archibald stayed in the hot seat until Durbridge replaced him and then I smashed Luke's time by 59 seconds. I knew as I took my place in the seat that I was keeping it warm for Ganna. I was pleased with my ride and had received a fantastic reaction from the crowd. Looking at Rohan, Evenepoel, Tony Martin, Stefan Küng, Victor Campenaerts, plus plenty of other talent to come, I felt a top 10 place to win Team GB that extra Tokyo spot would be a decent result, but desperately wanted better. Rohan stormed in, silencing all doubters with a brutally brilliant ride. A true champion. But of the others, only Evenepoel, Ganna and Paddy Bevin beat me, and with Filippo and Paddy it was by the slimmest of margins.

These were the biggest Worlds of my career. There was more riding on them for Team GB and for me personally than any other. We had a plan and I had stuck to it. A year on from the desolation of Innsbruck, I had come fifth, my best-ever showing at the Worlds. John Archibald's 14th place was a great performance by any standards, but especially considering he had had only a few days to prepare.

The TV cameras caught me in a long-held embrace with Chanel and Mum afterwards. Dad stood back, looking on with that small, modest smile of his that means he is very, very happy. Before they left me, Dad hugged me, with that extra little squeeze and a whispered, 'Well done, boy.'

I watched as he and Mum walked away, hand in hand.

Harrogate was rammed. Everyone there seemed to be enjoying it. In my interviews I paid tribute to British Cycling for putting 'a lot of eggs into the Alex Dowsett basket'. I said that it had come with pressure but that I had handled it. And I praised John Archibald.

John and I got on really well, had breakfast, lunch and dinner together for a week, sharing a lot of information about how we could help each other. That has always been the way I have conducted myself. Even though a time trial is an individual event, my teammate is my teammate and I want us both to do well. John was the same. We were both very open in trying to make us both go faster. I felt that we were similar people.

I stayed in Harrogate for a couple of days before heading back to Essex and did a podcast interview up there. The podcast was lengthy and we got to the subject of the Huub boys. I sang their praises, as I had always done, and said the only thing John lacked right now was a little bit of grunt. I backed that up and gave it some context by saying that at both the Nationals and now the Worlds, I had beaten the Huub boys but only just; that the way they were doing things was so methodical and successful that if they added a bit of World Tour nous to their armoury they would be unstoppable.

It would be pretty difficult to take offence at what I had said given the praise that filled 99% of it, but whoever was running the Huub boys' social media channel managed it. The podcast went live as Chanel and I drove south and Chanel watched social media light up about it. Their team account started an online tirade directed at me about World Tour riders and an insecurity complex and being afraid of the future. They posted pictures of me riding with my head up and taking the piss out of my position. Chanel messaged the Huub account to ask if they were seriously posting *crap like this* given that I had *nothing but respect* for John. They replied saying my comment about grunt was disrespectful.

Chanel put her phone away and said to me, 'Internet rubbish like this never gets solved with a tit for tat.'

'You're right,' I said. 'Let's go and talk it out like adults. Derby is on the way.'

John Archibald texted me to apologise for what the team was saying. *I'm sorry. That's not me.*

I know, mate, we're coming to see you guys.

The World Tour, as much as it's not liked at times and labelled elitist, is wildly competitive and does require a certain amount of power and toughness. That's the *grunt* I was referring to and the nous. Yes, the aerodynamics Dan and his entourage were obsessed with is hugely important and their knowledge of it is truly awesome, but you also need some of the brute power married to bare-knuckle fight that being on the World Tour gives you. That is what I had said in that podcast and that is what I explained to Dan, John and a few of the Huub boys in the reception of the Derby velodrome later that day. Dan said very little. He didn't agree with me and he refused to criticise his team's social media attack on me. It was a calm conversation and one that I found thoroughly depressing given how much I had admired them all. We agreed to disagree.

The call from Gary, my manager, came within hours of getting home from Harrogate.

'Israel Cycling Academy want you to stay.'

'Stay? I've never been with them. They turned me down.'

'True. And Cofidis have come in for you on more money than the Katusha contract, for two years.'

'Can I go?'

'No, not really, no. You have a contract and Israel have taken over that contract.'

'And told me they don't want me and that I can look elsewhere.'

'They've changed their mind.'

I sat down with Kjell Carlström, Israel Cycling Academy's general manager. We had been teammates at Sky and I knew him to be very dry and non-committal. (He reminds me of F1's driver Kimi Räikkönen.) He talked to me about the team and the project and he made it all sound pretty good.

'That all sounds great, Kjell. But I don't want to race for a team that doesn't want me. And you stated very clearly one week ago that you don't want me.'

'Didn't. We do now.'

'Why?'

He didn't blink. 'We didn't, but you just finished fifth in the World Championship, so now we do.'

Brutally honest. I suppose it's refreshing.

I could have said to him, *I don't like how you've handled it, I've got a better offer and I want to be free to take it up*. But I didn't consider Cofidis a better offer, other than financially. I respected Cofidis and would have been biting their hand off the day before, but I didn't see them as a team that would be progressively open-minded about the art of trying to go faster. On that side of things, I believed in the Israel project, backed by a billionaire with a self-proclaimed talent for racing bikes.

'Is there anything else you want to know or ask?' Kjell said.

'Yes, two things,' I said. 'One, I'm going to New Zealand for this winter. We're already in late September, everything's booked and organised. If you need me for anything, that's where you're flying me from. I also need to be back there for Chanel's admittance to the Bar.'

'Okay,' he said.

'The other thing is this. When I ride for Team GB I'm going to use what's fastest. If your kit isn't fast enough, I'm not going to be using it. Contractually, there is nothing you can do about it. It won't be branded, I won't make a big song and dance about it, but I'm on the road to the Olympics and shit kit is not going to get in my way.'

'Also okay.'

Israel Cycling Academy was formally admitted to the World Tour and changed its name to Israel Start-up Nation. ISUN eventually took seven riders from Katusha and I was one of the lucky ones.

I thought.

17

STAGE 8

Giro d'Italia, 2020

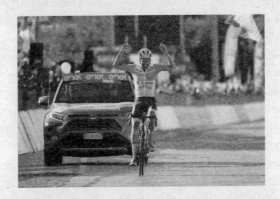

The 2020 UAE Tour was different to any previous races I had done in that part of the world, because I was now riding for Israel Start-up Nation and, with the boss and hierarchy out there with us, we had bodyguards and suburban SUV escorts with us at all times.

The first time the team owner spoke to me, I was standing with my Canadian teammate, Alex Cataford, and there were no introductions, no small talk, no asking us how we were – or even who we were. He just leaned in towards us and said, 'Are we respected within the peloton now?'

It was late February; the season was in its infancy and so was Israel Start-up Nation.

Alex replied enthusiastically that we were. Sylvan Adams, our owner, a man who had inherited his father's Canadian real-estate business and loved cycling, nodded, then looked at me.

I was more hesitant: 'Not yet, but it's getting better. We need wins to arrive on the World Tour.'

I was not ready for his reaction. He didn't look pleased. He glowered at me, then walked away. I immediately wondered if it was a mistake to offer an honest opinion to a billionaire.

———

Before we left the UAE, I got encouraging feedback from Kjell Carlström and one of the sports directors, Nicki Sørensen. I'd impressed not only with my riding but my ability to rally the troops and contribute to the team. I was on the early list of riders to be re-signed later in the year. That is music to the ears of any athlete over the age of 30, but within weeks the music had stopped and the world had fallen silent.

As soon as the pandemic hit, I got stuck into team lockdown activities, Zwift group rides and races, everything to help the team through the uniquely weird times. Along with Dan Martin and André Greipel, the three of us contributed to the team via our social media presence in a way no one else could.

The grind of five months under particularly strict lockdown in Andorra was transformed by the news, in April, that Chanel was pregnant. She got home one Friday afternoon from a hike and said she thought her period was five days late.

'Do you know what?' I said. 'I thought about that as you went out the door.'

'When have you ever been interested in my menstrual cycle?' she asked.

'Well, now,' I said. 'We're trying for a baby.'

'Fair point,' she said. 'Let's just wait over the weekend and see how things are on Monday.'

I was already holding the car keys. 'I haven't had my hour outside yet today. I'm going to buy about 15 pregnancy tests right now.'

An hour later, when she emerged from the bathroom, she didn't need to say anything. The look on her face said it all. I walked across and gave her a hug.

After that it was just a matter of goofy grins and not being able to concentrate on anything else.

Meanwhile, back on planet ISUN, I began to think more and more of that look Sylvan had given me when I said we weren't yet respected. I had good reason to wonder about it, given that I was watching my teammates getting re-signed for next year without hearing anything about my own contract. New contracts for the Canadians and Israelis weren't a big surprise, then it was Biermans, Würtz Schmidt, Rick Zabel, Van Asbroeck and Greipel – all good riders, but I was concerned. And slowly expecting a baby and facing a non-renewal of contract got my stress levels rising. I hid it at home, especially as by eight weeks Chanel was feeling like absolute shit.

'Early pregnancy is like being hungover without the pleasure of drinking,' she declared. 'And that's quite a challenge for a beer-wench like me.'

When Chanel was asleep at night, I'd lay my head on a pillow next to her tummy and listen to her breathing. I'd imagine the oxygen in her blood heading down to the life she was supporting and growing inside her.

Just keep breathing and growing my little darling, just keep going. I am so excited to meet you.

———

Around June of that year, rumours of Chris Froome joining ISUN were everywhere, and I got a call from him to ask about the team and the bikes. The TT bike was, if you recall, the Factor SLiCK that had arrived at my house before the Tour Down Under, ISUN's first race of 2020.

And it was, you might also recall, the bike Dad and I had stared at for some time when we took it out of the box, bemused – unnerved even – by what we saw. The SLiCK was big, with two parallel down tubes. I'd learned so much about aerodynamics since starting to work closely with British Cycling for Tokyo and this bike made no sense.

I was ready to be proved wrong. In fact, I was hoping to be.

I put it in a wind tunnel with my GB coach Michael Hutchinson.

It tested slower than what our opponents were on, cancelling out the gain from the Vorteq skin suit I had spent £5,000 on.

So, when Froome called me, I was upbeat with him about the team and honest about the bike.

'The time trial bike is painfully slow,' I said. 'I don't care how good you are over the next two or three years. You will not be able to win a Grand Tour doing TTs on that bike.'

On 9 July, it was announced the team had signed Chris Froome and that Factor would make a new time trial bike. Chris told me that he insisted on his contract that if Israel Start-Up Nation hadn't made him a competitive TT bike by March, he would be using his Pinarello.

Then I got a call from Factor. 'Alex, can you help us develop this new TT bike?'

I could feel myself instinctively going to respond, *Sure. I'd love to*. But, for once, I stopped myself jumping to help out. I had no contract for next year, I would potentially be helping produce a bike I'd never get to use, and Chris Froome was competition for Tokyo.

'You know what?' I said. 'The minute I sign a new contract with the team, I'll help you develop this bike.'

By late July 2020, when we emerged from lockdown for the restart of racing, my manager, Gary McQuaid, had sent half a dozen emails to Kjell Carlström, ISUN's general manager, about my contract renewal and about the possibility of me trying to recapture the Hour record.

The Hour was exactly the sort of high-profile success that would help ISUN, who had not won a race, start to earn the respect from world cycling it so craved.

Kjell had not acknowledged one of our emails.

I rode Strade Bianchi on 1 August and was the only rider from Israel Start-Up Nation to finish the race and then, at Tirreno–Adriatico, I excelled in the leadouts and got a tap on the shoulder from Quick-Step director, Davide Bramati, asking for my details. Although I got a message a few days later from Patrick Lefevere, Quick-Step's manager, to say the team was full for 2021, he had taken note of me and this glimpse of a dream scenario (to team up with Alaphilippe, Evenepoel, Asgreen in the strongest team on the World Tour) was a nice reminder that it was still possible to feel good about cycling.

In the time trial on the last day of Tirreno–Adriatico, on the Adriatic coast, I had problems early on with the handlebars slipping and then I stopped halfway through when the bars came apart completely. I took a good long look at the clear blue sky and told myself not to scream and not to kick the shit out of the bike. I knew I could not afford to continue the race. To finish 20th in a contract year, and look like you're trying, is worse than limping in last. Last place tells everyone something's gone wrong; 20th looks like you're not good enough.

For the World Championships in Imola in late September, I was the only rider in the top 10 not on team kit. I changed up all the equipment with only aerodynamics and speed in mind. I borrowed the frameset from my friend Symon Lewis at Specialized and had to block out the logos. I bought the Shimano Groupset myself. The front wheel was from Harry Walker at Revolver. The saddle was one that Team GB had developed. It looked like an instrument of torture to the untrained eye but was a dream to ride. The helmet was given to me by Poc and the rear wheel I borrowed from my performance chef, Alan Murchison. (To be clear, Alan is loads of top athlete's performance chef; he doesn't live with me.) The difference between my set-up and the ISUN set-up was 30 watts, which is huge.

I thought that Imola would be a turning point, that surely now Kjell and Sylvan would see the situation for what it was and move heaven and earth to fix it. Israel Start-Up Nation had not only taken over Katusha's licence, they had inherited the kit deficiencies too. In plain sight at the Worlds, I had put in a poor performance to come ninth and still beat an ISUN teammate, Matthias Brändle, who rode better than I did but was on the Israel Start-up Nation set-up. I had done 50 watts less than Matthias and beaten him by a minute and a half.

Because of the kit.

For a brand-new team on the World Tour, who desperately wanted to be accepted by the peloton, this was useful information, vital intel, a golden opportunity to transform your results with a kit change.

———

As Chanel's pregnancy progressed, we were told that to get the proper support she would need to go to Barcelona for the birth. There was a risk that if the baby was female she could have a lower clotting level and so be at higher risk of bleeding. We both agreed that if we had to go to Barcelona, we might as well go to the UK and be at home. She moved back in September. I went with her and took an hour out to visit my old friend, Andy Lyons. We had a heart to heart and I admitted how scared I was by the contract situation with my first child on the way.

'Mate, I think my career's over.'

On 27 September, as Chanel entered the final trimester of the pregnancy, I received an email from Kjell.

Dear Alex,

As per regulations, we hereby need to send this letter to whom we don't intend to renew the contract at this point of time.

Best regards,

Kjell Carlström.

I turned away from my laptop screen and felt the life drain out of me. I walked to the window and looked out at a featureless autumn day. The cloud was low and I pictured my flight tomorrow, my plane disappearing into the clouds and emerging into the blue, heading for the land of the Azzurri, the country that had been the setting for such key moments in my life. For the first time ever, I would take on the very particular demands and challenges of the Giro d'Italia with no sense of hope or of really, truly, being a pro cyclist in a pro team any more.

We are about to start a family. My partner has suspended her entire career for mine and will now do so again to have our child. Just when she needs me most, to step up, to provide, I am out of a job, possibly out of my profession.

I am 32 years old and I'm fucked. I'm pathetic.

The regulations Kjell's email referenced are the contractual obligation of every UCI team to inform their riders by 30 September if they are going to re-sign them.

Three days after his email that spent me spiralling into the wormhole, on that UCI contract deadline day, Kjell called me to shoot the breeze. He paid me some compliments on how well I had led out in Tirreno and said he hoped I could do the same at the Giro. Then he got down to business.

'So, Alex, we had to send the email but that doesn't absolutely mean we won't re-sign you.'

'Then re-sign me. You know we're expecting a baby, right?'

'Yeah.'

'You've been dangling the *maybe* of a new contract since February. I'm going to the Giro as demoralised as I possibly could be.'

'Okay.'

The team asked me to help with pre-Giro adjustments to make the Factor Tractor (the riders' name for our TT bike) as quick as it was ever going to be. The directors also asked me to take the team meeting ahead of the prologue. I agreed to do both these things but found the team's schizophrenic approach to me totally depressing.

I arrived at the Giro in a place I'd never known, the point of no longer believing I could win. It wasn't the same as the anger that had swept me to Commonwealth Gold in Glasgow. In some ways it was the opposite, the lifelessness caused by stress and having the carrot of a new contract dangled in front of you by your masters, being asked to lead while being told you were not wanted. Everything was going to feel different about this Giro. Instead of it being the first Grand Tour of the season, in spring, the COVID-affected calendar meant we would ride into autumn.

Geraint Thomas was a race favourite. Nibali was looking for a third maglia rosa. Simon Yates had won Tirreno–Adriatico and Jakob Fuglsang was also looking strong. The team's focus was on the Tour de France with André Greipel and the Vuelta with Dan Martin, and we were in Italy to make up the numbers. Not a single conversation or article about the race would have mentioned Israel Start-Up Nation, still winless in any stage race or event. No one saw the Giro as the place where that would change. I knew I couldn't compete in the time trials due to the bike, so Matthias Brändle and I decided we would race each other for fun and to gather data to show other team managers what we could do. On different kit and in a different state of mind, I would have been straining at the leash at the prospect of taking on Rohan Dennis, Filippo Ganna and Victor Campenaerts in the three time trials, but instead I feared that helping out with the bike fit and giving the team talk were the most useful contributions I would be making. But even as I chose my words for that team talk, I had a feeling that racing in this state of mind – not so much carefree as beyond caring – might at least be an interesting experience.

And there was something else. Touching down in Italy, sucking in the atmosphere in Palermo, I realised that for this country, which had taken the first heavy hits of the pandemic when it reached Europe, this event was a rebirth for more than just the Grand Tours. This was a huge moment for Italy. I needed to remember that. To start back at the beginning. Lucky to be alive. Lucky to be riding a bike for a living, if not for much longer. Blessed with a baby on the way.

Be 16 again, Alex. Just get on your bike and pedal fast.

In the race manual, a journalist called Pier Bergonzi, who understands and loves the Giro as much as any person, quoted Gandhi:

Life is not about waiting for the storm to pass, but learning to dance in the rain.

I did nothing in the first time trial and the team rarely featured in the break in the first week. On the morning of Stage 8, I tweeted,

I just cleaned my teeth before drinking my coffee. I hope the rest of the day goes better than it started.

On the team bus, Matthias Brändle sat next to me and peered over at the route map I was studying. The finish had a climb with the potential to derail the sprinters.

'Perfect day for a breakaway,' I said.

He nodded. 'Uh-huh.'

The coaches gave us a talk and said it was a day off from tactics. 'This is a breakaway day. We've got a bunch of riders that can do breakaway stuff, so go and do breakaway stuff. Don't overthink it.'

The first 100km out of Giovinazzo were flat and twisty along the Adriatic coast, and very hot. The second 100km were more punishing with two categorised climbs.

I went with Matthias in an early breakaway. There were six of us in it, we started rotating straight away, working hard and opening up a gap. It was perfect to have Matthias in there with me, but there was a hell of a long way to go. The other four riders were Simone Ravanelli from Androni and Joey Rosskopf with CCC, another rider who was fighting for a contract. Joey could climb and he could TT. Matthew Holmes was in his first year with Lotto–Soudal (now Lotto–Dstny) and was well suited to the climbs we had ahead of us. And Salvatore Puccio, who had been a work horse for INEOS all his career.

The main obstacle of the day was a 10km climb in the middle of the stage. I was worried about it because I knew that if the others wanted to attack on that, Matthias and I would be in trouble. But we pretended we were doing the break a favour by riding the front, when actually we were just setting a pace we wanted to ride at rather than the pace they wanted, and that way we got over the summit together with a 14-minute gap behind us to the peloton.

All of a sudden, this felt pretty interesting.

My chances of winning this had just gone from 1 in 160 to 1 in 6 – but actually to 1 in 3 because it didn't matter if it was me or Brändle.

Down the radio came noises about the peloton making a move, but soon after we heard Nicki Sørensen say, 'Okay, it's all calmed down now behind you and this breakaway will be going to the finish line.'

I looked at the other five.

There is no reason why I shouldn't win today, I told myself. *I can be the guy that does this.*

I went through it in my head. I am not on the TT bike, so I have a good bike underneath me today. I have the aero helmet on and a lot of these boys do not. I have aero socks on and I have a real fast skin suit that I had made by Nopinz. (The team suit didn't fit, wasn't aero, had given me saddle sores and was now in the bin.)

I have done everything to prepare and I can win this.

That's what I was telling myself.

Brändle and I were tucked in on the drops. Every time we got to the front, we'd lift the speed. We'd do so with less power because we were both tucked in small. We were trying to chip away at the other four without them quite knowing it, using less power than they thought because we were so committed to a strict aero position, and so that the others would think *They'll pay for it later* – and not be right.

Nicki came on the radio telling me and Matthias to attack with 60km to go.

'Mate, it's early,' I said.

Matthias and I got close and had a chat.

'How do you want to win this?' he said.

'I need to have no one with me,' I said. 'I need to be on my own ahead of everyone. What about you?'

'I can beat all of these guys at the sprint,' Matthias said.

'Cool. We got a good two options here, mate.'

I attacked first. It was always going to be chased down, but it loosened things up and that was our intention. The race within the race had begun.

I saw the next climb, puffed out my cheeks and admitted to myself, *Oh this is steep. This is a proper climb*. Everyone rode hard. I sat in behind Holmes, Puccio and Rosskopf, who were pushing confidently. Suddenly, we were not in my territory any more but in theirs, where aerodynamics wasn't going to help me and a bit of grunt was required.

I started to struggle. I started to doubt myself. I looked into the wormhole. *This looks terrible*. Two teammates in a breakaway of six and they both get dropped. At the top of the climb, I was in no man's land, losing ground on the front three. But then Brändle came screaming up to the back of me with Androni behind him.

'Alex, let's go!'

Quickly, we worked together, back on our territory, we launched straight back up to the front three. They were surprised to see us and looked at each other for answers.

Nicki came on the radio. 'You need to do something now while you got them on the back foot.'

Brändle opened up a 10-metre gap.

I shouted to him, 'Do it! Go!'

He pressed. The other riders reacted and shut him down immediately.

Nicki screamed, 'Alex, you gotta react!'

I hesitated. I second-guessed myself for a split second. In my mind, there was still 18km to go and that last climb. Then I blocked out all the thinking and attacked.

I knew I had to do two things. First, hit them with so much speed none of them wanted to be the one trying to bring me back when they were saving themselves for the end. Second, stay in the saddle. Try not to look like an attack. Going hard but staying down. On this occasion, on this day, in this particular moment, I did both perfectly.

When I went, how I went, the others looked at me but didn't react, because I wasn't igniting the panic created by Brändle's full-on attack. They had just shut Matthias down and they didn't want to go do it again. They wanted someone else to do it.

Matthias came down the radio; 'Go, go, go, Alex!'

Then he went on to the wheel of whoever was going up front, kept stealing second, disrupting any coherent effort by the others to come back at me. That's when my gap skyrocketed and we heard Nicki going:

'That's 15 seconds. It's 23 seconds. It's 32 seconds.'

I slung my hands over the bars, puppy paws position, and used every ounce of aero to build the lead.

Nicki said 'It's 52 seconds, Alex,' and I started thinking, *What the fuck are they doing? Don't they know I'm pretty good at riding by myself?*

The final climb before the finish at Vieste was pure pain; my thighs burning, my heart and lungs screaming; and my mind taunting me with the possibility that I could win this, like the man on a rooftop who fears wanting to jump more than falling, the possibility that I could screw this up when all I had to do was not crash.

That climb sucked the life out of me and my lead was cut from 50 seconds to 25, but as soon as I got over the summit I started to rebuild the gap. I was powering on and it hurt so much, but I knew that you come out the other side of pain and that knowledge almost makes the pain not exist. And, suddenly, with 3km to go and a 40-second lead, I understood they couldn't catch me. I ran the numbers in my head, the gap, my speed, theirs. They had run out of road. That small breakaway I had got myself into so long ago, it had never been caught, and the race within the break, I was winning it.

This was mine.

Then Nikki came down the radio. 'Alex, have a think about how you want to celebrate this because you've won this stage of the Giro.'

But I couldn't think about that even though, as a kid at the Academy, we'd sometimes practise celebrations as we rode, emulating heroes, saying how we'd do it if we won. All that went out the window. I didn't know what was going through my head. It was a kind of disbelief and an overwhelming surge of emotion.

I could feel Chanel watching, Mum and Dad too.

Come on, Alex! I told myself. *For them. For the baby. To put food on the table. Everything depends on this.*

Into the home straight, my mind turning over the immensity of what was happening, I saw a limping dog appear ahead of me on the course. That's not a cycling term or a euphemism. There was a small dog running on three legs down the home straight towards the finish line. A tradition in Vieste? A symbol of good luck? I had no idea; I just needed to avoid the thing. The dog headed left, so I went right and it struck me that if that dog swerved now and took me out, that would have summed up the year perfectly.

And I was so petrified of being caught still, even though I knew it wasn't possible, that I was still gunning it. Then I could see the line at last. I had a little look behind me just for my own sanity and security to make sure there was no one there. I finally sat up. I took my arms off the bars and didn't really know what to do with them, ending up with my hands in front of my face. Then I held on to my helmet. It felt totally unreal. There was, I guess, an element of ferocity to how much emotional energy I had pent up in me. I jabbed my index finger in the air, grinning demonically. And then I clenched my fists and punched the air with joy and relief.

- I had just saved my career.

———

Chanel had gone out. There was no reason why she would have been watching a stage of the Giro which wasn't a time trial. But as the volume and regularity of messages bombarding her grew –

This is massive!,

This is happening!,

'Come on Alex!!! –

she rushed home to see what the fuss was about. She sat at the kitchen table watching on her phone, because the TV had not yet been connected. And she told herself, repeatedly,

He's not going to do it, he's not going to do it.

Attagirl.

She did this for two reasons: in order not to get her hopes up and because she had never heard of me winning a road race. It's not simply that she hadn't seen it happen in the four years she'd known me, she hadn't heard anyone raise the concept of it ever being a possibility.

As the commentators grew more sure that I was going to win, she asked Albert, our cat: 'Is this actually happening?' and all the while, she insists, the baby was kicking and kicking. When I crossed the line, she bawled her eyes out.

Then she headed over to my parents' house and joined them and Lois, who was also pregnant. They all sent messages.

> *I'm in bits*, from Dad.
>
> *I've aged*, from Mum.
>
> *I've gone into labour*, from Chanel.
>
> *I've gone into labour*, from Lois.

(They hadn't.)

When I rang Chanel, all I could hear was her sobbing down the line. I joined in. I would later discover that Andy Lyons was standing in his living room watching with tears streaming down his face. Alan Murchison had abandoned a training ride and returned home and was leaping and screaming around his living room, still wearing his helmet, pausing only to send wildly happy messages to Chanel. From that small straw poll, everyone who knew me went to pieces. What a lucky man I am to have such friends.

To say it was joy would be underselling it. To say it was relief would be underselling it. To say it reignited some confidence in myself would be nearly right, but not quite. I didn't suddenly feel confident, but I felt happy. It was huge. Because I had come to believe over the previous months that my winning days were over.

And although I struggled to keep it together afterwards, I was, at the same time, very aware of what I was saying in the interviews. That is not to say it was planned, but I knew I had things to say and an opportunity, at last, to say them. As the cameras trained on me, I was proud to not have a single piece of Israel Start-Up Nation kit on my body. The socks and skin suit I had paid for myself having first researched them for aerodynamic gains, in a way that my team were simply not doing.

I described Matthias Brändle as instrumental. 'If he wasn't in the break with me,' I said, 'there's no way this would have happened.' I thanked Nicki Sørensen and the guys that were at that race. I made sure not to mention Israel Start-Up Nation once in any interviews, just the individuals in the team who supported me. I said that it had been a tough time. With my voice breaking with emotion and my face looking as genuinely bewildered as my bosses had been making me feel for months, I told the media, 'I've got a baby on the way in January and I don't have a job currently for next year. I needed this so badly I don't know what my future holds.'

It made for horrible viewing for ISUN. They put up a load of great content about the win on their social channels, but were met with a barrage of *Give the man a contract*. It wasn't the response their historic first win on the World Tour should have got; I made sure of that.

The reports described the race as a 'tactical masterclass', but I'm not capable of them. What it was, however, was two teammates who had a great instinct for each other and respect for each other, and every minute of work and thought I had put into aero and all the kit I had bothered to go out and source for myself, the engine I had developed over many years and my time trialling skills plus a real, live, deep, pulsating fury at how my bosses had discarded me. It was all those things disguised as a masterclass.

When I turned in that night, Alex Cataford was asleep on the other bed in our dingy hotel room. Bloodied gauze, plasters and tape covered eight major injuries on the left side of his body that he would now have to carry through the rest of the race, starting with 208km in the mountains the next day. We've all been there.

That small, bare, yellow-walled hotel room summed up professional cycling. One man lying awake, his heart and soul bursting with happiness at being a winner, daring to hope that the day ending had won him a contract that would mean he could support his family. Six feet away, another cyclist lying broken and in pain, with every ounce of courage, strength and the madness that we all have to possess to do this about to be called upon to get him back into the race tomorrow.

This was Alex Cataford's first Grand Tour. He was an absolute gentleman to room with and made me the coffee of my dreams in the morning with his

Aeropress. Stage 8 had been horrible to him. He'd crashed and skinned himself as badly as I had seen in a long time. He would carry on for another four stages until a cold, wet day when the team had to pull him off the bike because he wouldn't stop riding despite being in so much agony he had become delirious. My team had to carry him into the car and take him home and, with the pain getting worse, to hospital where they would discover he had been racing for four and a half days with a broken hip.

Alex Cataford – the team you ride for still had a long way to go back then to earn the respect it craved, but you were already there, you amazing, kind, tough, lovely bastard.

I lay in bed and replayed the race in my mind. Chanel had worried that it looked like I was giving ISUN the middle finger as I crossed the line. I really wasn't. I wouldn't. And I realised something blindingly obvious and of no significance to anyone on the planet other than me. Both my Giro stage wins, two of the greatest moments of my cycling life, had come on Stage 8. It is the eighth stage of the blood-clotting process that I lack. It is the synthetic Factor VIII I take which allows the blood to clot and me to ride a bike.

8 has been good to me. Thank you, 8. You are officially my favourite number.

———

On the rest day, two days later, Sylvan Adams joined us for a ride and came alongside me.

'We'll talk about the future later today,' he said.

There was a team meeting scheduled for 7 p.m. and I had to do a bucketload of interviews that the team's press officer had organised.

Before the first one he said to me, 'Alex, I think you mustn't talk about your delicate situation.'

'Go on, what situation is that?'

'Well, the situation around your contract. It doesn't make the team look good.'

'I've said everything I need to say,' I said. 'I'll be nice. But if someone asks me if I have a contract, I'm telling the truth: that no one from the team has breathed a word about a contract still.'

Kjell finally messaged me to say we'd meet at 6.30 p.m. That meant we would have 30 minutes for the whole discussion about my future. It was just Sylvan, Kjell and me. The first thing Sylvan said was, 'Your win was a fantastic team effort.'

'I couldn't have done it without Brändle,' I said.

'We've let you down,' he said. 'We've waited far too late to do this contract. It's been a strange year. We want to keep you. We value you as a rider. Next year, we want to give you more responsibility in the team. We want you to help develop the new time trial bike and be a road captain in races.'

That took the wind out of my sails.

'Thanks. Thanks for owning up.'

Then he said, 'I'm going to make you an offer. We're going to make you the same offer as most of the other riders are on.' He said a figure.

It was just over half what I was on.

'That's absurd,' I said. 'I have just won this team's first ever Grand Tour stage. I just made history for this team. You want me to do more work next year on top of riding, for nearly half the money.'

'I'm going to give you a bonus for winning a Stage at the Giro.'

'Tell you what, keep the bonus and pay me the same as I'm on now.'

He knew that my back was to the wall. I knew that I was going to sign a contract that meant I could support Chanel and the baby and me for another year or two.

'It's irrelevant anyway,' I said, 'until we talk about the Hour record, because actually that's far more important.'

'What Hour record?' Sylvan said.

'The one that I've sent numerous emails to Kjell about this year and received no response to.'

Kjell spluttered, 'But, Alex, but, but . . .'

'It doesn't matter,' I said. 'What matters is, it's happening. It's exactly the sort of thing that would have helped put your team on the map, Sylvan, but you've blanked me on it, so I'll do it independently.'

Kjell went to speak, but Sylvan spoke over him. 'Can I suggest you do it next year at my velodrome in Israel?'

265

I said, 'The Sylvan Adams Velodrome [for that is its name] hasn't got walls. It's got a roof, but no walls, which makes it a non-starter for an Hour record. Anyway, I've been asking Kjell to reply about an Hour record for months and now I've got a team meeting.'

Which I went to.

I wasn't deluded I knew I had absolutely no power in this negotiation. But if people treat you like you don't exist, it is really not a good idea to encourage them by rolling over. Not immediately.

A week later, on 19 October, the second rest day, the three of us had another meeting scheduled. On my way to it I received a call from Chanel. She was in Chelmsford hospital. She had gone in for a routine check at 28 weeks and developed palpitations, with a resting heart rate lying down of 165bpm. They had admitted her to a ward with suspected sepsis.

'I'm coming,' I said.

'There's not much you can do,' she said. 'They won't even let you in 'cos of COVID.'

'What does it mean?' I said.

'I'm hooked up to an IV and they're pumping in some heavy-duty antibiotics.'

'The baby?'

'It's no worries. They're monitoring everything.'

She didn't tell me at the time, but they had said matter-of-factly to her, 'If there's continued problems, we'll just take baby out.'

'Alex, I know this is hard for you to hear, but it's important for you to stay there and sign a contract, finish the Giro. We need it. You do that and I'll do this.'

I took a moment to think. It was Chanel who was going through it, and it would actually have been the easiest thing to quit the Tour and rush back. That would have seemed like the great gesture on my part, but in fact I would have been running away. It would have added to Chanel's worry about our future and achieved nothing. If I needed to be there, she'd tell me.

'Okay,' I said. 'You do that and I'll do this. I love you.'

There were six stages remaining and on every one of them, Tao Geoghegan Hart, who was on track to win the entire Giro with INEOS Grenadiers (and did so) asked me in the bunch how Chanel was doing. Every single day. He genuinely cared. I've never forgotten Tao doing that and being a winner simultaneously.

Minutes after my call with Chanel, I sat down again with Sylvan and Kjell. I had spent the whole week angry at their offer but now my mind was elsewhere.

'You said to me last week that you want to pay me 100K, which is what you pay most of the riders on the team.'

'Yes,' he said. 'The market's changed.'

'You asked me to help develop the time trial bike and to be a road captain next year. You're asking me to do more than all of those riders that you want to pay me the same as. So, for the bike riding bit of what I do, you actually value me less than them. I can't work for someone who undervalues me and thinks I'm lesser than the rest.'

'What do you want?'

'I named my price and Sylvan agreed to it.'

We on shook that. I have rarely disliked two people as much as Sylvan and Kjell. Given how they treated me, I have to presume the feeling was mutual. And when me signing a two-year contract extension with Israel Start-Up Nation was announced, this is what Sylvan and I said for the media:

Being on the road with this team is great fun. It's clear Israel Start-Up Nation is one of the most exciting up-and-coming teams. I'll be playing a loyal supporting role to the sprinters. When your teammate wins, you feel like it's a win for everyone.

Alex made history by winning Israel Start-Up Nation's first Grand Tour stage. But as importantly, he's a great teammate, with leadership qualities that motivate and guide his fellow riders. He is truly appreciated by his teammates and the management of our team.

I nearly wet myself reading it.

I left that meeting and went to my room. I lay on the bed and waited for a call and hoped and hoped Chanel did not have sepsis and that the baby was okay. She called after a half hour that felt never-ending.

'I'm in the clear. They're going to keep me in for two days and monitor me. They don't know what caused my heart to go crazy, but it's not sepsis.'

I stared at the ceiling with a big smile on my face and an aching to be beside her.

'What's your news?' she said, brightly.

I told her we were back in business with ISUN for a couple more years. We didn't kid ourselves we were ecstatic about being with ISUN. It was a case of needs must.

'You either get put back in the stable or you get sent to the glue factory,' Chanel said. 'You're back in the stable. Well done for biting your tongue.'

I laughed.

'I miss you,' I said. 'I'm sorry I'm not there for you.'

'I do wish you were here,' she said. 'It's lonely.'

'You're doing so brilliantly.'

'You too,' she said. 'Won a race and got us a contract.'

'It was nothing,' I said.

Then there was silence, the silence of longing.

'Don't worry about your boss,' she said.

'You're the boss,' I said.

———

Chanel and I went it alone in setting up a fresh assault on the Hour record, which was now held by Victor Campenaerts. The UCI backed us and we went out and started to get sponsors, with no commitment and little interest from ISUN. The attempt was set for 12 December, 2020 at the Manchester Velodrome. I would be returning to the scene of my 2015 triumph. Bradley Wiggins sent me a personal message wishing me the best of luck. He said I was looking really good after the Giro and my stage win there and that he would be watching. It was really nice. I don't know what effect retiring and other changes in his life had on him, but as a fan of his and as a racer who always looked up to him, I think finishing his career was good for him. At various times I've had reason to consider him a tosser, a genius, and one of the funniest blokes out there. He's bitched at me and he's been supportive too. That's competitive life for you. That's what the Academy taught me to handle. I wasn't expecting that message and it was a nice one, which I appreciated from the man who earned the right to be called Britain's greatest ever cyclist.

One month out from the attempt, I got COVID and was advised to postpone, something that I did reluctantly with training having gone so well. But in the bigger scheme of things, it was easy to get over the disappointment because four days after Christmas our daughter was born. Healthy. Noisy. Beautiful.

A few days later I got a message from Paulo Saldanha, the team performance director at Israel Start-Up Nation, saying he'd like to talk. He called at 10 p.m. that night. I presumed he wanted to either congratulate us on the baby or discuss the upcoming training camp.

'Alex, there is a reason I have called you. I'm really disappointed in you.'

'Right.'

Suddenly, the glue factory didn't seem so unappealing.

'I'm disappointed with what you've been spreading to the team. A bad, negative energy.'

'You're going to have to elaborate, Paulo.' I thought I was the guy who kept the morale on the team up. I thought I was one who made sure they were all okay out on the road, who fitted their bikes for them, fetched water for them, raised their profile with a Grand Tour stage win.

'You know you've been telling everyone the TT bikes are shit and you've been telling everyone the power meters are shit.'

I thought about it for a second and said 'Paulo, yes, you're right. I have been doing that. And, yes, there's probably a better way to have gone about it. I am sorry because that's the last thing I actually want to do. The people in this team I care most about are the other riders, so I actually feel really terrible if I've created a bad vibe. For that, I'm sorry.'

He said, 'Okay. Thanks Alex. I just have to be honest.'

'But we're going to talk about this, Paulo. If you're going to call me up at 10 p.m. and not congratulate us on having a baby because you just have to be honest, then can I honestly tell you how I feel in this team?'

What ensued was a 30-minute monologue; no shouting, not even a raised voice, minimal foul language, just a non-stop flow of grievances that I had no idea was going to come out, about how I had been treated and, after that, about the kit.

'Everyone knows the power meters are bad. It's talked about openly. Shouldn't the riders know the TT bikes are bad too?'

'I don't know what you mean.'

'Look at Alex Cataford, bucketload of power, good aero position, we know the helmet's good, skin suit is okay, he works hard and cannot crack a top 50 result. Shouldn't he know the bike is bad rather than wondering what's wrong with himself?'

There was silence.

'We've got a TT bike Ganna could not win a race on. I've got a power meter where nobody trusts the number that comes out of it, not even you lot. What have I got to sell to other teams? This team has single-handedly stopped me being a cyclist. I'm not a cyclist, I'm certainly not a time trialist. I have nothing to sell to any other team. It's like your boss taking away your laptop and your data and your testing gear, handing you a notepad and pencil and saying: "Do your job better, Paulo." I finished ninth at the Worlds on anything but this team's kit, and you can see from Matthias' numbers that he shat all over me in terms of power output, but I beat him easily. Surely you can see then that something is inherently wrong if I'm just hopping on to a Specialized and finishing top 10 in the Worlds with an average ride and Matthias can't crack a top 30 with one of his best-ever rides.'

'I've always fought for you, Alex.'

'Fuck lot of good it's done. And why are you making this call, then? I went to the Giro with a letter saying we're not going to re-sign you and a phone call to say that we might. I've just become a dad and you're toying with me.'

'I didn't think that was right, how they treated you. But can I say something, please?'

'Of course.'

He said nothing for a bit, then he sighed and said, 'Well, Alex, well, I think it was a mistake to re-sign you.'

'I'm getting mixed messages from you, Paulo. You just said you fought for me. You're all over the place.'

'You just seem really bitter about it.'

'Bitter? Paulo, in the January team training camp you made all the riders do a full-tilt time trial in 5° the day they'd seen their TT bikes for the first time. It was stupid and asking for a load of injuries. Some of these kids have never had a TT bike before. I took it upon myself. I messaged all the guys individually to say, *if anyone wants a bike fit, I'm happy to do it*. Paulo, I missed every massage and coffee break on that training camp to bike fit 12 of my teammates because you didn't have the foresight to do it yourself. I did that. Now, if I was bitter, if I didn't think there was a future in this team, do you think I'd have bothered with that?'

Paulo said, 'I called you to give you a bollocking, but actually on behalf of the team, I feel like I need to apologise to you because that's not right. You've not been treated right. I don't understand it.'

That interested me; that this man clearly did not know what he thought; that he seemed to be battling internally with what he had called to say. *You're a troublemaker, Alex. I'm sorry for how they treat you. You're bitter. We all owe you an apology.*

And nothing changed. At the 2021 UAE tour, the power meters were all over the place yet again, leading me to overcook my ride and blow my doors in the TT at a time when every TT was an audition for the Olympics. Many of us felt that our careers were going down the drain. Riders in the peloton referred to ISUN as a shitshow. That's what they would ask us: 'Is it the shitshow everyone says it is?'

When work is stressful, home becomes a haven, and you yearn to get back to it. With a newborn baby there, those feelings only get intensified.

Time at home in Andorra with Chanel and our daughter was a balm on the strains of life with the team. Our daughter would tend to settle into a deep sleep in the early evenings as the sun went down and the mountains cast shadows across the valley which then crept up the slopes and enveloped the town. Glowing orange lights would appear as the daylight faded. I would stand at the window with my sleeping baby girl in my arms, absorb the solemn privilege of parenthood, feel the gentle rise and fall of her breath, watch the expressions ebb and flow across her face and watch the sun bow out and the peace of the mountain silhouettes.

The apartment was snug and calm. Chanel and I would tiptoe around our sleeping baby and communicate in whispers and smiles. We would settle into long, silent embraces and cuddles on the sofa, sometimes let the apartment fall dark around us. The peace was magical, life speaking for itself. The tenderness in that space was everything that work was not and could never be. It felt safe.

It felt wonderful.

And so, as if we couldn't bear too much of a good thing, Chanel and I decided to ruin it all and reschedule that attempt at the Hour.

In Mexico.

18

WINNERS AND LOSERS

The Hour, 2021

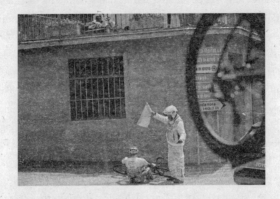

There are pros and cons to attempting to break the World Hour record.

The cons first. It hurts. It becomes an obsession. It takes over everything. It changes your body shape into the time trialling equivalent of a large potato. It costs you every minute of your time and, if you go it alone without the backing of your World Tour team, a lot of money. It's fucking miserable. It's the Death Star of self-doubt and loneliness. It hurts way more than you think I meant when I said it hurts.

The pros – or the pro. You might become a part of sporting history.

But it's not really about weighing up the pros and cons. If the thought of it is lodged in your head and it won't leave you alone, then you can write as many for and against lists as you like, chew it over, take other opinions on board but essentially, none of that matters.

Because you're totally screwed.

And left with only one consistent thought to which you keep returning. That to live with regret when you have a say in the matter is a mistake.

Jackie Joyner-Kersee, one of the greatest athletes of all time, said, 'It's better to look ahead and prepare than to look back and regret.' Chanel told me, 'The Hour is still in you and you'll kick yourself if you don't go after it again.'

In what possible time or universe would it be sensible to ignore those two women?

The Hour was an itch I had needed to scratch since I broke it in 2015, in part because of how comfortable the first record had felt. That is not to say that it didn't hurt, but I knew I could have gone faster, further, through more hurt, and not come undone. Another reason, if I am honest, was that I had held the record for such a short length of time. Just five weeks after my triumph in Manchester, Bradley Wiggins surpassed my 52.937km with a brilliant ride of 54.526km in the London Velodrome. In so doing, he joined giants of the sport like Merckx, Induráin and Coppi in having taken both the Hour and Tour de France.

And then there was another fundamental reason. Despite having matured into a leadout man, I am a time trialist first and foremost and, while I learned in 2015 that the Hour is different to a time trial in some important ways, rather than being the ultimate incarnation of it, it remains an undisputable fact that if you have the mind and body of a TT specialist, the Hour sits there as a permanent fixture in your thoughts and teases you and beckons you and sometimes drives you crazy with temptation, all the while kidding you that it isn't so bad after all.

So, a bit like Tinder, really.

But unlike swiping right, the Hour was unfinished business in my life.

I saw my chances of breaking it as 50/50 – no better, no worse. And although I knew that going it alone, without the support of a World Tour team, would be tough, I also knew that it was the greatest remaining opportunity for me to raise money and awareness for Little Bleeders and the Haemophilia Society while I was still on the World Tour – given that, and I don't want to shock you here, I was not going to win the Tour de France.

Chanel took on sponsorship and all the groundwork, the biggest and toughest chunk of setting the attempt up. It was an enormous undertaking and one she had to do without the wonderful Taryn Kirby, who had been instrumental to the COVID-cancelled attempt the previous December but was now living in Australia. The pitch deck Chanel created set out the coverage sponsors would get from backing the event. Pfizer immediately committed half the funding – £50,000 – or what we thought at the time would be half. They wanted to support us without being the title sponsor, because they didn't want it to look like a Pfizer event and didn't think we would want that either. I have a viewpoint on pharma companies that most people don't share. In my mind, what I have sitting in my fridge, keeping me alive and active, is down to a pharmaceutical company. If they didn't have a business model, they'd have no incentive to make it, they probably wouldn't make it and I'd likely be dead by now. Pfizer's immediate support for the Hour was what made Chanel and me go for it. It probably, also, made us think it would be easier than it was.

We were a team of eight. As well as Chanel and myself, we had my agent, Gary, who was instrumental in putting it together and dealing with more team politics than is healthy. Michael Hutchinson was the entire coaching, performance and engineering team. Alan Murchison did the food, but that doesn't begin to touch on his contribution as chef, nutritionist, assistant mechanic, assistant travel agent, raconteur and lifter of spirits.

Simon Lillistone was our listed manager; meticulously organised and calming, he took the event by the horns and set us on our way. Chanel credits him with saving her from a nervous breakdown. Which one, I'm not sure.

Mark Coyle was our broadcast logistics specialist, although in our small band of committed, generous people no one had titles and everyone pitched in wherever needed. When it came to TV and broadcast, the UCI set a burdensome load of minimum requirements in the contract, one of them being that it had to be a broadcast event. Mark was the guy who managed to find a production company in Mexico which could deliver all the broadcast and photography, then achieved the coup of getting the event broadcast live on the BBC TV red button. Chanel had set about finding Mark the day I suggested I do all the TV and broadcast stuff using my smartphone. We would have been all at sea without him.

The eighth member of the team was our daughter, who was fast approaching her first birthday. It started as a running joke in Mexico, all of us saying that she was a crucial member of the team. But it became a simple matter of fact; without her, it would not have been half as much fun. Mentally, I might not have made it to the start if she hadn't been there lighting up our lives every day.

The Haemophilia Society were massively involved too, by facilitating payments and holding the funds from sponsors, something we couldn't do.

My job was to ride the bike, fast, in circles, for 60 minutes.

———

The Manchester velodrome was unavailable. It was having a new roof put on. London was not the surface I wanted to factor into the equation. My thoughts turned to Aguascalientes, in Mexico, where Victor Campenaerts had set the record. It was fast and at altitude and I lived at altitude.

Between Wiggins breaking my record and Campenaerts breaking his, there had been ten unsuccessful attempts and three of those, by Tom Zirbel, Martin Toft Madsen and Dion Beukeboom, had been in Aguascalientes. I was in regular contact with Victor, and with Ashton Lambie, the individual pursuit specialist who had competed in the 2018 Pan American Track Cycling Championships in Aguascalientes. I had been listening to both of them talk about Mexico for a while.

'Let's go there,' I said.

It was a wise decision in cycling terms, but would heap on extra layers of stress. The fact that it was touch and go whether I break the record was neither stressful nor surprising. There are no world records on offer in sport which don't involve putting your neck on the line and taking risk. Records are, by definition, an attempt to do something never achieved, and that is a step into the unknown. The stress came from neither the odds nor the unknown but from the logistical demands of setting it up without the backing of a Grand Tour team. And that was worse than I could ever have imagined, even though Michael Hutchinson warned me that was exactly how it would be.

Michael is a fiercely intelligent individual, an academic as well as a brilliant coach and an outstanding cyclist in his day. I have always looked up to him. He worried profoundly about the stress on me of organising the attempt negating the marginal gains he could find for me in training.

'There's no such thing as a non-physical stress,' he told me and Chanel, more than once. 'You have to factor stress into the marginal gains, as a loss.'

We listened, knew he was right, but we never did factor them in. We couldn't. Chanel and I just took the stress on board and hoped it didn't matter. We had two separate evenings where we realised we were tens of thousands of pounds short, having already put that amount in ourselves, and unable to put in more. For a period of weeks, we woke up every morning too scared to check our inbox because every day there were new logistical nightmares and unforeseen obstacles. Everything kept mounting up. We were only five people going to Mexico, but we were taking 14 bike boxes full of equipment. Every waking hour that was not spent training was spent meeting the social media and branding requirements of the sponsors, building the bike, dealing with Mexico. It was incessant.

Inside those bike boxes, along with a lot of other stuff, was the Factor HANZŌ time trial frame, HED Volos wheels, Vittoria Pista Ora 23mm tyres, an AeroCoach Aten 61T golden chainring and AeroCoach Ascalon aerodynamic handlebars. That was my set-up.

The low point came with a mistake we made when booking the flights to Mexico. We spent a sizeable chunk of the budget on flights to Mexico going through Fort Worth, Texas and then discovered that, because of COVID, no one could travel through the States in transit from Europe. Nothing in the booking process had stopped us doing just that. We were despondent, until British Airways responded to a tweet I put out and came to the rescue. But the flights issue was going to come back to haunt me again soon enough after Israel Start-Up Nation didn't respond to our warnings that I would not be allowed on to the return flight they had me on for the same reason.

There are plenty of elite sports teams out there which are a rich man's toy. Only some are successful. Most of them are a great place to be if you're in favour and a misery if you're not. The events that unfolded off the track during my second Hour attempt taught me that ISUN probably never wanted to give me a new contract after my win at the Giro but felt obliged. Consequently, they were never sure how to act when, after they blanked my Hour ambitions, I decided to go it alone. They did put in £15K in the end, were the only sponsor to pay after the attempt, not before, and the only sponsor to be unhappy with their coverage.

———

Chanel's days were filled with looking after our baby, talking to sponsors and delivering branded track boards, vlogs and social media posts. She had to block out two hours of my time every day to produce the content required.

'Alex, you need to not be doing this,' Michael reminded me.

I just shrugged helplessly.

'I know,' he said. 'If you don't do it, there is no Hour. I know. But it's a loss on the track.'

'I understand,' I said.

The Hour is about stress, but also obsession, because it is not only about the marginal gains that bring down the amount of power required from you, it's also a constant search for ways of producing that power. It's obsessive because every single thing in your life becomes analysed as a potential gain or loss of power. Everything you eat, how you move around, whether to go to bed at 9 p.m. or 10 p.m. Everything comes under the microscope.

And in my search for gains, there was nothing more consuming than the skin suit.

When Team Sky started talking about marginal gains many years ago, Michael and I were both in the camp of riders who thought, *Yes, that's clever and makes total sense, that's brilliant* while the other camp thought, *Get a life*. Mexico was the coming together of all my years of education in and appetite for the aerodynamic gains to be had on the bike and from the skin suit.

Unlike many, I had been through the process of developing skin suits from scratch and seen for myself the gains to be had from having the fabric oriented at the right angle and seams in the optimum place. When I finished a wind tunnel session, I would go through the numbers with the engineers and designers and

be part of the decision-making. This degree of involvement is a strength and a weakness, the latter being that if something is not right it consumes me.

We had battles with Vorteq, the skin suit supplier, because the gains that they thought they would find didn't materialise in the tunnel. They were head and shoulders above anyone else in the field, but that came at a premium – namely £14,000 for one skin suit. To produce them, they made a 3D print of me for wind tunnel testing. I witnessed my legs being 3D printed, showed Mum and she nearly passed out.

Vorteq were confident of delivering a 5% gain and delivered 3% on a best endeavours contract. All that money went on R & D, not on guaranteed results. They were pissed off that I was unimpressed. They are brilliant engineers, but their customer relations left a bit to be desired and with my money in their bank account they refused even to deliver the suit to us. For fourteen grand, I'd expect a skin suit to be flown to my door on the back of a spangly unicorn, but Michael ended up collecting the suits from Ellis, a Vorteq engineer, at Rothwell services on the A14. Exotic stuff.

The stress of it all took precisely the toll that Michael had predicted. In training, I was hitting numbers, just, but it was a fight. I would find myself staring at my laptop in the early hours of the morning, trying to source from somewhere in the world 8mm bolts for the bike that were light enough to give me gains but strong enough to hold the bike together under extreme duress. More than once, I walked exhausted into the kitchen to find Chanel there in tears at the impossibility of what was being asked of her.

In amongst all of this, Chanel's Grandad in New Zealand died suddenly from a stroke. It was devastating for her. She had lived with him for a small part of her childhood and the two of them were close. Unable to get back to New Zealand due to the border closures there, our mission on the bike left her with no time or emotional space to process her loss. Even the livestream of the funeral eluded her, taking place as it did when we were mid-flight to Mexico, and she was left with calling her family as soon as we landed to 'be there' for the wake. By the time we arrived in Aguascalientes, we were both flat and mentally exhausted.

Michael felt a lot of responsibility. It was all on him from a coaching and numbers point of view, although he did have the ever helpful and hugely knowledgeable Billy Fitton and Laurence Birdsey at British Cycling double-checking some of the numbers. In the week of track training we had in Aguascalientes, day 2 was encouraging, what Michael would call a 'cheery day'. CdA (a unitless measurement of one's efficiency for overcoming aerodynamic drag) dropped and power required reduced to 336 watts. Michael told me the provisional numbers as I got off the bike and I said to him, 'I think I can do this.'

I was aware, however, that Victor Campenaerts had two months in Aguascalienetes to prepare and he had also told me that his good training days were usually followed by a few bad ones. Sure enough, next day, my power required spiked to a very unwelcome 360 watts and I couldn't hit it. Variations in the aero package like this aren't unknown. They can come from the power meter. They can also be real – for example, taking a suit off and putting it on again can introduce significant differences depending exactly where the seams and wrinkles end up sitting, and the tension in different bits of the fabric, since they're all designed to function at their best at a particular stretch. The outlier was day 2 but human nature latches hopefully on to the best results and places faith in them.

The good day was reality. The bad days are a glitch. That's what you tell yourself.

On practice day 4, I did 20 minutes of race pace with full race protocols around it and produced adequate numbers. I noticed that in the empty stadium was a middle-aged man alone in the seats, watching everything we were doing. The manager of the velodrome told me that he had been a local cyclist of some repute until he suffered a serious head injury. The man watched intently, barely moving, not an expression crossing his face. When I finished, I went up into the auditorium, introduced myself to him in my basic Spanish, and sat with him. He seemed happy to have company, so we spent 20 minutes together talking within the limits of my language skills. We shared one-word observations about cycling and the velodrome. He wasn't old but there was a frailty in his voice, and a sense of his body having been broken, which moved me profoundly. When I said goodbye to him and got to my feet, I heard his thin voice say my name.

'Alex Dowsett . . .'

He nodded at me and then nodded at the track and smiled.

'Si, si, Alex Dowsett. Vamos.'

I don't know why it's stuck with me, but it has. By the time the whole experience of the Hour in Mexico was over, those calm, softly spoken moments of hesitant Spanish and careful listening to what he had to say had become important, even if now I can't put my finger on why. Moments of stillness are rare in life, rarer still that week in Aguascalienetes, and I was grateful to him for that gift. I hope he knew we were talking cyclist to cyclist, not cyclist to spectator.

The roof of the Aguascalientes Bicentenary Velodrome is held up by a column of air being blown permanently upwards by a large fan on the in-field. When the air is switched off, the roof descends gently on to the arena. Maria, our Airbnb hostess, discovered that if she put a balloon in the air stream it would fly up to the roof and this became a game to delight our daughter.

Maria, her husband, Leonardo, and their son, Javier, became a part of the team. We ended up employing Maria to look after Juliette at the Velodrome during the day and Leonardo to drive us back and forth as we had one hire car but way too much kit to fit in it. They became invested in the attempt, wearing Hour record polo shirts every day and doing everything possible to help us and make us feel welcome. It was a very special bond with them that built up that week.

There was a pool at the Airbnb. Alan wouldn't let us go in it because he turned out to be the Marvel equivalent of a health and safety inspector, protecting us from evil, food poisoning and waterborne bacteria with the slogan *You're not going in that fucking pool*, which we heard every day when we dared even to look at it.

Every evening we all sat around the large kitchen table with our laptops. Michael and I analysed the numbers and what to change in the set-up. Chanel and Mark were doing the heavy lifting of meeting sponsors' and broadcast requirements respectively. Juliette played with us and around us. Alan would appear with bowls of amazing food, which he'd put down in the middle of the table between the laptops. The atmosphere was brilliant despite everyone's fatigue. The whole team got on brilliantly and knew their own responsibilities. There was never a cross or harsh word spoken in that house.

At night, Chanel and I rewrote the rules of romance by sharing pillow talk about budget deficits, our liability, commitments to sponsors, our daughter. We spent many of the daylight hours in the garden filming content. Observing this one day, Michael said to Alan, 'This is what will kill him. When he should be resting, having a bite to eat, having a chat about something else, playing with his daughter, he's doing all this. If he misses out, it will be down to this.'

'It certainly won't be down to my food,' Alan said.

The day before the record we arrived at the Velodrome to find all the sponsors' banners going up, the UCI installing themselves and the Tissot timers setting up. That was a pressure moment. The moment I stopped kidding myself I was the Robin Hood of the Hour record, secretly in Mexico with my small band of Merry Men and Women, about to steal it without anyone noticing. It was a reminder that a load of sponsors were expecting me to deliver and hundreds of thousands of people would be watching. It wasn't Robin Hood, it was David and Goliath, but did I really know who, or what, my Goliath was? The Hour? ISUN? The rest of the world? Myself?

Chanel and I sat by the pool together that evening while Alan, always sensitive to our needs sometimes even before we were, looked after Juliette inside, delighting her with his play, his chatter, his voice, his animated expressions exactly what a toddler loves. All so that Chanel and I could have a quiet moment together. The same way that other couples would lie by the pool and feel the heat beat down on them, so we lay there, eyes closed, hand in hand, soaking up the pressure.

We called the stadium manager to remind him to set his alarm to switch the lights on at six in the morning, so that we were at 28°C (82°F) by the start, as the lights were the only source of heating inside the arena. Then we turned in.

The next day was 3 November, 2021. I was 33 years old and it was six years since I had broken the Hour record with a distance of 52.937km. At 10 p.m. UK time, with family, friends and cycling fans watching back home and all over the world, I rode 54.555km, significantly further than my first Hour record, further than Bradley Wiggins had gone.

And 534m less than Victor Campenaerts.

I had failed.

———

I started well but after 14km found myself two seconds off the record pace. I pulled some of that back and remained within a second of Victor for the next 20 minutes. I never felt comfortable, but it felt like a ride I could keep thrashing out even though it didn't feel good. But I couldn't. Normally, the lack of fizz in my legs, the lack of clarity in my head, means that tanks are being drained and the conviction I can soldier through is going to prove an illusion. At 30 minutes, I felt in control and that I could do it. At 35 minutes, that had changed and I started to lose control of my rhythm. My pace slipped and I couldn't get back on top. I had the will. I was psychologically ready and willing to push myself through any sort of mental darkness, but I was empty. In the last 20 minutes, lap times drifted up towards the 17-second mark and when I sent the signals to my body to power up and hit the 16.3 seconds that I needed, there was no response – or, at least, no immediate response. And so, even though I regained speed in the final 20 laps and started to outpace Victor's record, the damage had been done – and I knew it. I lifted myself momentarily out of the aero position, perhaps in acknowledgement of defeat, before returning to work and pushing hard right up to the Hour. The emptiness I felt as I freewheeled to a slow gradual halt is something I never want to feel again. The fight was gone from me. I was jelly.

Chanel and Michael helped me off the bike and led me to a chair. I could not have walked unaided. My body no longer belonged to me. I had the extraordinary realisation that, in this moment, there did not exist a position or manner in which to place my body which felt okay. Everything hurt, physically and spiritually. It was painful to merely exist. Never had I understood more the truth that the Hour exposes you like nothing else. It had cleaned me out.

As Michael helped me down on to a chair I muttered to him, 'It hurts to sit, it hurts to stand, it will hurt to lie down.'

'Ah,' Michael said, 'that's exactly what Chris Boardman said after one of his attempts, so we did it right.'

I was interviewed soon after, holding my daughter on my lap, and my voice sounded like an old man's. I sounded like the man I had seen sitting in the red seats watching me train and with whom I had spent those lovely, calm minutes talking. I felt a stabbing sorrow that I had let him down, but I knew that wasn't true. In my faltering voice, I said, 'Everyone believed in me, I believed in me. And this was as far as I can go. I'm proud of that.'

54.555km was the third biggest distance in the modern history of the Hour record. (Now, at the time of writing, it is the fifth.) There is clearly no need for shame.

It would be a while before the colossal disappointment and feeling of failure really hit me. Initially, strange though it may seem, as I clawed my way back from the twilight of emptiness and exhaustion, my first coherent thought was of admiration for Victor and for Dan Bigham, because this pain had been earned by riding a shorter distance than they had. Sometimes as a professional sportsperson you just do have to stand back and admire the achievements of others. And if I had been capable of standing, that's what I would have done.

Instead, I mustered the physical and emotional strength to say this to the media:

> There were three targets coming into this. The first was to break the record. I came up short. I want to take the chance to say well done to Victor and to Dan Bigham because there was a World and British record up for grabs today and I was a bit shy of both. But today was still a success because the other two targets were to see how far I could go, and 54.555km is as far as I can go and I'm proud of the distance that I managed to cover today. But the most important point today was the awareness that we've brought to haemophilia. The overriding message for young haemophiliacs, anyone with a

rare condition, anyone who is facing any kind of adversity, just give it a shot, because the biggest failure today would have been not to have tried.

Michael's reflections were more specific: *I'm absolutely confident that if he hadn't had the stress of setting this all up, Alex would have broken the Hour record in Mexico today. He was very, very close.*

———

The next day, 4 November, we sat in the small airport of Aguascalientes. I was physically and mentally spent. The relatively sunny disposition I had shown in interviews and for my YouTube channel earlier in the day had deserted me. I could barely raise my head.

It is safe to say, I was in a dark place.

Chanel, Juliette and the team were flying to Mexico City and from there home to London. We had fulfilled all the YouTube and social media obligations to sponsors. I wasn't ready to hear it at the time, but Chanel and Mark had already received bucketloads of generous feedback from them for the attempt, for how close I got, and for how we had met all their requirements. They were proud to associate with what we'd done and the raising of haemophilia awareness.

The one thing preying on Chanel's mind, and what was left of mine, was ISUN's insistence that the flights they had booked for me to Israel via the States were okay when we knew, from our experience of coming out to Mexico, that US immigration would not allow anyone to fly through the country if they had been in Europe in the previous two weeks.

My flight opened first.

'You're not going to be able to get on this flight,' Chanel said, not for the first time.

She was desperate to keep me with the rest of them, given how down I was. I went to check-in. The man behind the desk was ready for me.

'Alex Dowsett?'

I looked down and saw that he had a note in front of him with my name on it.

'Yes.'

'Yes, you can't get on this flight.'

Fatalistically, I smiled. 'Yeah. Thought so.'

I explained the situation.

'I'll happily call Homeland Security but *they* called *us* to say that you are not getting on the flight. I'll call them again to double-check.'

'Thank you.'

The call was over as soon as it began. 'Yes, you're not getting on this flight.'

I rang Gary in London, 'Mate, I can't get on this flight.'

'Of course you can't.'

It was almost 24 hours since my world record attempt and there had been no word from Israel Start-Up Nation apart from a voice message from Kjell to Gary saying how disappointed Sylvan was by ISUN's coverage as a sponsor (all of which had been signed off by Kjell himself) and adding that it was down to me to sort any ticketing problems and get to the team camp in Israel.

The flight to Mexico City that Chanel, our daughter and the others were taking was full and the one after that got into Mexico City too late for me to get an onward flight to Tel Aviv. I was not physically in a state to do a 10-minute drive up the M1 let alone hire a car and drive five hours across Mexico. Chanel and Alan looked at flights from other airports, trying desperately to connect the dots to get me out of Aguascalientes even if it meant a string of domestic flights. They worked frantically, looked into buses and trains to the capital, anything to get me on a plane with them to London so that I wasn't stranded.

Then it was time for Chanel and the team to get their flight to Mexico City. They said their goodbyes and I watched my wife walk away with my baby girl. I sat alone with my bike and felt about as low as I can remember in my life. And, I would later learn, as Chanel turned back to wave a final time, she saw me sitting among my equipment, crying. I don't mind admitting to that. I had just failed to break the Hour record. I was physically drained. I knew that a team I had long felt unsure about seemed to actually hate me. I suddenly felt very young and very alone.

I faced the choice of spending three days like this by myself in Aguascalientes, waiting to reach the 14 days since I'd been in Europe so that I could fly to Israel via the States, or missing the team camp in Israel altogether – something that I knew would be the final nail in the coffin of my relationship with the management.

When I finally spoke to Kjell, I told him that Chanel and I had put more of our own money into the Hour than Israel Start-Up Nation had, and now he was telling me to pay for flights because they had booked the wrong ones.

'I thought you were making money out of this thing!' Kjell said.

'No! It was for charity!'

We came to an agreement. I would pay for a flight to London, and ISUN would pay for my flight from there to Israel. But there was still the issue of being stranded in Aguascalientes, or as I came to think of it that day, Kjell-on-earth.

I called Leonardo.

'Hola, friend,' he said.

'Hey, Leonardo, I'm in trouble. I need to get to Mexico City.'

Half an hour later, Leonardo's son, Javier, appeared at the airport to drive me through the centre of Mexico from Aguascalientes to Mexico City.

An angel.

We set off and I called Chanel. 'I'm in a car with Javier. It says we'll be there in five hours and 20 minutes. It's too tight, isn't it?'

'I want you on this flight with me,' Chanel said. 'I'll book it. Just get here.'

'Can you get $500 out of our account to give to Javier?'

'Yes, of course,' Chanel said.

'No, Alex!' Javier said.

'Yes, Javier!'

Of course there were flights to London the next day. Of course there were hotels in Mexico City airport where I could sleep until then, which was probably what my body needed most. But, dejected, depressed, drained, my desire – my need – to get on that London flight and spend eight hours with Chanel and our daughter close to me before I returned to ISUN became existential.

It was one of the most stressful journeys of my life, because for the whole way we were on the limit of the boarding gate closing. I sat there with the Waze app telling me our ETA was three minutes after the gate closes to two or three minutes before the gate closes.

Javier drove as fast as he could and all my beaten-up mind could think was, *Fuck you, Kjell, for doing this to me.*

Over the next two hours we fell adrift of the ETA we needed at the airport, a little more every few miles, until we were 10 minutes down, and had to accept that we weren't going to make it. Just as with Victor's record, the attempt was slipping away. I wound down the window, rested my head and felt the wind blow against my face. I let go of the possibility of making the flight and basked in the release of no longer hoping. I was sick of racing against the clock. I just wanted to shut down and stop caring. The breeze felt good and the air was warm and I fell into a strange sort of state which wasn't sleep but was deeply restful, almost semi-conscious. And a memory came to me, as we hurtled across Mexico, in a battered-up old car which was about as far as possible from the private jets and helicopters sometimes used for flying riders from race to race, a memory I had long ago lost. As the warm air beat against my face and I stopped worrying and stopped thinking, I found myself returning to one of my first ever races. It appeared incredibly vivid in my head, the sort of memory that starts playing like an unscheduled movie in your mind and you just sit back and let it roll.

I was in a VW campervan with four other guys being taken up to the Junior Tour of the Peaks. It was 2005 and I raced for a local team, Glendene CC. I was 16 and I had never taken part in a race at this national level. The Peaks was one of the biggest junior races of the calendar. It was also the hilliest. Bob Downs, our coach, drove us around the course and I got carsick because it was so hilly. There were five of us, and Glendene had four sets of carbon-fibre wheels and one set of aluminium wheels.

'I don't stand a chance here,' I said to Bob. 'This is beyond anything I can manage. Give me the metal wheels, let everyone else take the carbon, because this is beyond me.'

Bob said, 'Okay, but it doesn't matter if you can finish or not. Just enjoy it.'

I want to be like Bob Downs when I coach or mentor juniors. Everything he knew, all that he had achieved, was distilled down to an ability to make you get on the bike and enjoy yourself. He never banged on about what he'd done (you found out from others that he had won Gold at the Commonwealths and been to the Olympics), but he put it all into making you fall in love with being on the bike.

The Peaks that year was four laps, roughly 60 miles in total. I got in the early breakaway without having a clue what I was doing. I was just riding. With a lap to go, on instinct, pure feel, I attacked the breakaway. I don't know why I did it. I didn't know how to race bikes and none of us knew if I was any good, but I went away on my own and when I got to the finish line no one had caught me. I thrust my hands in the air and when I brought the bike to a standstill, I hugged my dad and burst into tears.

I hadn't expected to see the finish line, let alone cross it first. I was continuing to surprise myself. I was beginning to realise I was not going to live the life of a sick boy. Bike racing was happening to me, without me knowing much about what it was. So much of professional cycling is about control and targets and tiny margins, but the Peaks was simply about pure innocence and joy, pedalling as fast as I could and seeing what happened. Not saving any effort for later, everything was in the now.

Reliving that race as we drove across Mexico was like an out-of-body experience. I could taste the tears on my teenage face and a feeling surged through me, the same way I use to feel anger, but this was joy. That had been proper bike racing without the politics. The Peaks was happiness. That was the time I discovered I was good before I felt the pressure of it.

Alex, I told myself, *don't let today cloud the fact that everything that has happened since the Peaks has been a wonderful ride. Even this failure in Mexico has been a blast.*

You've got to be in it to win it. But sometimes, just being in it is sublime.

And perhaps that is what tells you that your time is up, when you find yourself overwhelmed by the memory of a boyhood win years ago and the suspicion that professional cycling is not going to make you feel that good ever again.

We made up time to the airport just when I had stopped hoping or caring. We were back in with a chance of making it. Chanel made the gate aware of my late arrival and with the help of Javier, I was suddenly that mad-looking Englishman dashing through the airport with his bike in tow. The airline people were waiting for me, ready to check me in, take my stuff and get me through.

As we took off, I watched the ant-like cars on the labyrinth of double-decker highways in the spawl of the city, and thanked Javier again in my mind for giving me these extra transatlantic hours with Chanel and my daughter.

———

When I landed in Israel and switched on my phone, waiting for me were the messages that had started to flood in, forwarded to me by Chanel, from the Haemophilia Society, from Mark and Simon, voices from the real world beyond ISUN, thanking me for the effort, praising the time, saying what it meant to people from the haemophilia community. I went on to the YouTube livestream link and scrolled through the reams of positive messages and saw the fundraising was going up and up.

All the sponsors were messaging too:

So proud to be part of this event, Look at that awareness you've raised for haemophilia. What a great effort.

I'm not convinced I deserved the praise, but I felt better than I had.

I joined up with my teammates in Israel for the training camp and next day we went to Sylvan's velodrome, and there was a crowd of kids there. All the team sat down to talk to them. It was great and, hopefully, inspiring for everyone. It was very relaxed, hanging out with these young people and chatting.

Sylvan said to a group of them, 'You know, Alex is a bit different because he's just done an Hour record and he's actually the only professional cyclist that has haemophilia.'

He looked at me. 'Yes, that's correct isn't it? You're the only haemophiliac in professional cycling.'

I said, 'No, I'm the only haemophiliac in professional sport.'

He went quiet, in a totally un-Sylvan way, like he was almost taking on board something that had been said to him.

'Really? Okay.'

And the moment passed and we all moved on, but it stuck with me. And I look at it as a stupid waste, how little he and I got on. For a brief moment he had seemed to allow for the fact that he had a gap in his knowledge. I think it registered as interesting to him, maybe even as a lost opportunity.

As we sat with all these kids who would be inspired by his visit and helped, I don't doubt, by his philanthropy, and as the money and increased profile poured into the cause of helping young haemophiliacs, did any small part of him think: *What if I had picked up on Alex's Hour attempt more than I did, and on his life story, his cycling journey with a rare disease, and put my name to that, funded it, taken the stress away so he'd beaten it? I would have been the guy who made it possible for the only haemophiliac in elite sport in the world and his charity to break a world record. And he would have been wearing Israel Start-Up Nation kit and logos and branding?*

As I look back at the fact that I stood up for what I thought was right or fair during my career, and that I spoke up about the things which I believed were stopping us from going faster, I think now that it was possibly a bad thing at times. I'd like to think it was a good thing for the most part, and I can say genuinely that it was always done with the right intention. But it made me seem like a pain in the arse at times, too. I wasn't always right, not by a long way, but I always spoke out in the interests of going fast or in the interests of fairness. It's true that I was guilty of putting my hand up to say, 'We are going to win fewer races because of this,' but it is equally true that I would offer to give all my time, energy and knowledge (once I had acquired some) to help improve the set-up for the whole team.

I've never been apologetic for being that guy, because it was always in the interests of performance, and we are elite athletes doing what thousands would love to be able to do, and it's such a waste of that honour not to put everything legally possible into going faster and being better.

Because it is over oh so quickly.

As the days passed, I began to feel okay about my attempt. 54.555km in an hour is a distance that now makes me proud. I gained consolation from telling myself that I may want to be a hero to my daughter, but you don't have to be at the top of a leader board to be a good father. I'd rather do it from there – of course I would, because I'm ambitious and vain – but it is not what's going to matter to her. I think of how much I love my dad and him being my hero, and my dad does not mean what he means to me because of his trophy cabinet, it's down to the man he is. And the one person who matches him as my hero is Mum and she doesn't have a trophy cabinet.

So, I began to feel okay about coming up short in Mexico.

The biggest failure would have been to have never tried. I said those words to the media when I got off the bike and as the weeks passed I began to truly believe them.

In Israel, I got a message from Dan Hart at the London Hospital:

All of us who try hard and fail, that's what life is all about.

Like the roof of the velodrome at Aguascalientes, the cause of haemophiliacs will need continued pressure to keep it where it needs to be. That's down to me and although it does not come naturally, public speaking is one of the ways I can and must advocate for greater haemophilia care to enable young sufferers to participate in sport and have a better life. One of the key messages I share is the importance of not being afraid to fail, of trying without any guarantee of success. It's a message that resonates with everybody I have the privilege of meeting, from sufferers of rare diseases to the corporate crowd.

If I had broken the Hour for a second time, gone two for two, then I would have been more celebrated, more pleased with myself, but possibly less relevant to the people I have a duty to help. I would have had to bridge a larger gap between what I had achieved and what youngsters with haemophilia or their parents think is possible for them.

Maybe it was supposed to work out like this. Maybe I had one last bit of changing to do, to be a better, more useful, advocate for haemophiliacs than I was. Maybe if I had broken the Hour again, I would have just stayed the same.

Change is good. But it doesn't mean you get to write the script. That's where the risk lies. Change can feel like the moment when you fall from your bike and, momentarily, everything goes into slow motion and you wonder: *How bad is this going to be?*, only to land softly and brush yourself down. I was a different person when I took the Hour record in 2015. I know that simply means I matured and that's kind of mandatory in life. I'm not asking for a medal for doing some growing up over the years, but I am realising that the Hour when I failed was the greater achievement.

19

BORN LUCKY

Leaving the World Tour, 2022

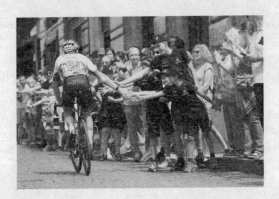

I wake in the early hours from a dream about a tunnel. I am cycling through it in pitch blackness. I can hear my bike cutting through the cold tunnel air, the echoes of my exertion, but I am blind.

I check the bedside clock. It is 5 a.m., late enough to be worth getting up and starting the day. All is quiet in the apartment. My wife and daughter are asleep. I tread silently to the kitchen and make coffee.

The tunnel was real, and it is not the first time I have dreamed about it. It lies somewhere between Pizzo and Praia a Mare on the coast of Southern Italy. I rode through it at 65km/h on Stage 11 of the 2018 Giro and it was so badly lit that the middle section was blackness. I could see spots of light from a couple of Garmins and Di2s and that was all. I have rarely been more terrified on a bike than in those 10 seconds of coffin-like darkness. I knew not to accelerate or decelerate. Your chances of survival are highest if you maintain the exact trajectory and hope to hell that everyone else does the same. It helped that nearest to me was Tony Martin.

'That was terrifying,' he said, breathlessly, as we emerged into the blinding daylight.

We went back to the commissaire car that follows the race.

'That tunnel was unacceptable,' Tony said.

'I know,' the official said.

'What the hell do you mean, "I know"?' Tony said.

'It was really bad,' the guy said.

I said to him, 'If you're not governing this, who is? Who is responsible for this?'

He shrugged.

Things like that happen far too often on the World Tour. When Tony retired in 2021, he said, 'I just didn't feel safe in cycling anymore.' With a year to run on his contract with Jumbo-Visma, his exit was a damning indictment of safety in the sport and how the UCI and ASO fail to take it seriously.

'I started fighting for this a long time ago,' Tony said, 'and what I can say now is that nothing changed.'

———

As I make my coffee, a thought comes to me, the realisation that I was wrong when I once said that being signed by Team Sky was a way of giving haemophilia the middle finger. That was my attitude to the obstacles placed in my way by being sick, but it is not how I think about my disease. Not at all. It is something that is integral to me and that I love, because I have no wish to hate anything about myself or to swap my life out for one without my disease.

There is plenty about myself I am critical of, but there's no way I feel negative about my haemophilia. It has given me the life I have had so far. It put me in a swimming pool and then on a bike and that ended with me riding in the Tour de France, winning at the top level, travelling all over the globe. It made me part of a community of sufferers and clinicians I love and admire. It has taken me on the ride of my life. Without haemophilia, I would never have had a professional sports career.

Without haemophilia, I would have been another average footballer.

It is sometimes hard for me to fathom what has happened in my life so far. I would pinch myself, but I've had so many skin fold tests that I'd rather not. But one thing is clear to me.

I was born lucky.

From the second I arrived in this life, delivered with the use of forceps that could have caused a severe haemophiliac baby like me irreversible brain damage, but didn't, my luck was in. The delay in my transition to preventative treatment saved me from being one of the many who lost their lives in the contaminated blood scandal. I remember being back home for a few days in 2017, between the Tour of Romandie and the Hammer Sportzone Limburg, and watching a *Panorama* programme about the scandal, the two thousand British people given a death sentence by their treatment, the thousands of mums and dads whose lives are forever wrecked by loss, the adults who still today are discovering they have Hepatitis C from transfusions in their childhood. I sat staring at the blank screen long after I had switched it off.

Would I have found cycling even if Dad hadn't gone windsurfing that evening on the River Blackwater and met Eric Smith? Maybe I would have seen another bike and taken a shine to it, but without Eric and Glen Smith there wouldn't have been Steve China taking me on and coaching me. Without a local man called Colin Cleminson losing a close friend and wanting to create something in his honour, there would not have been the Glendene Juniors cycling team for a few years. That was a moment in time and I chanced into it; the sort of timing and good fortune that gives me shivers to think how easily it might not have happened. Between Bob Downs at Glendene and Steve China, I received an education as a junior without which I would not have had a career.

What fortune was it to fall into the orbit of a teacher, in Robin Bevan, who not only loved cycling but raced? A man who grew up worshipping Pantani and was crushed when the world learned that his hero had cheated; a man who introduced me to the British Cycling Academy; a man who is now head of a secondary school where one quarter of his pupils cycle to school, a phenomenal achievement. He has done more for cycling in this country than I have.

How different would my life have been if a cyclist called James Millard hadn't written me a race plan to win the Richmond Grand Prix in Yorkshire – one that got me, a 20-year-old, a phone call with Axel Merckx, who took me to Livestrong?

James Millard was three or four years ahead of me in cycling, but never got on to the Academy. But when I was watching my hopes of a pro career going down the drain under Max Sciandri and I went back home to get looked after by Mum and take part in the premier calendar race Axel Merckx had never heard of, I called James and said, 'I don't know British racing at the moment. If I want to win this race, how do I go about it?'

He talked to me for an hour and dictated the script for my race.

'Try and get in the early break. Your biggest disadvantage – that you are by yourself with no teammates – can also be your big advantage. Once you are in the breakaway, if any teams have more than one rider in the break, do no work whatsoever, just sit on the back.'

I did exactly what he said. A few riders in the break made comments to me, telling me to work. I ignored them exactly as James had instructed. I rode like a *see you next Tuesday*. There was a reshuffle on the climb, and John Tiernan-Locke and I started working it because James had told me to. More riders arrived in team multiples, so I stopped working and went to the back of them and Wouter Sybrandy criticised me: 'You should be working this.' I ignored him. I attacked when James had told me to, with 40km or less to go when there was a crosswind or tail wind or on a climb if I had the legs.

'Don't make your attack obvious from the front, Alex, come from behind with speed.'

Winning that race got me into Livestrong.

It was the race where I got laughed at on the start line for wearing a skin suit and silenced those deriding me. If James Millard had not sent me a script for the race, a transcript of our hour-long conversation, there's no way I would have won it, not a hope in hell. I've surpassed James as a cyclist so many times in so many ways, but I still look up to him to this day, and this book would be unfaithful and incomplete if I were not to place him here in it – along with Andy Lyons – as one of the greats in the cycling universe from my perspective. I learned more about racing tactics in an hour with him than I had done in my entire time at the Academy.

I have always been lucky.

———

I walk across to our living room window, taking my coffee with me. Coffee is a big thing for professional cyclists. If you're experiencing difficulty getting to sleep, ask one of us about our own coffee-making regime and play the reply back to yourself at bedtime.

I watch the first hints of daylight above the mountains, a deep blue creeping into the night sky. I will miss the sight of these peaks when we return to England. We wake up here to the sound of a river. I will miss that too. People here can walk to the ski runs. I am finally free to learn to ski and have done so this winter with my two-year-old girl. It's fantastic here, but soon we'll head home.

We've made some good friends in Andorra. One of them, Mike Woods, recently asked me to name my career all time high and low.

'You can only have one of each,' he said.

If it's limited to one, then it's relatively easy. The Stage 8 win at the 2020 Giro, for proving to myself that I am still an outstanding bike racer. The low was how it felt to ride for Israel Start-Up Nation and the way I became smaller every day that I belonged to them. Simple. In Mike, I was saying this to someone who has a good relationship with ISUN and its owner. He and I respect each other's differing experiences there. We appreciate that people are affected in different ways by the same thing.

Dan Hart discovered something similar when he found some people in the haemophilia community saying to him, 'Please don't talk to us about that bloody cyclist again.'

For some, I am the last role model they need. We took that very seriously and asked, *How should Dan and Little Bleeders use me and my story to help sufferers without overwhelming them with a feeling that being a haemophiliac professional sportsman is amazing – and amazing doesn't apply to them?* The challenge is to talk without alienating non-athletes for whom it will be incrementally beneficial to exercise and lose weight, within realistic boundaries. That's why discovering in Mexico that trying and failing meant more to some of the haemophilia community was such a revelation.

The work we do must have impact. When I was in Mexico, I had asked Dan to get involved in a LADbible haemophilia awareness campaign. Dan was in Gozo delivering a lecture when he got a message from a friend telling him that the LADbible campaign got six million views in the first few hours. (It was soon nine million). Dan called me.

'Alex, my lecture that evening was to a hundred people,' he said. 'If I write an academic paper about haemophilia care, I'll be lucky if two people read it.'

We were excited. It was eye-opening for us. We've got to learn how to reach people. Severe haemophilia remains a devastating diagnosis despite medical advances and the need to help normalise life for sufferers is of paramount importance. A lot of children still suffer from being too protected or under-treated. Little Bleeders must also keep looking for new disadvantaged individuals, those with non-severe haemophilia who aren't a priority for early treatment and, consequently, live back in a less-advanced time. And what about girls who have their own challenges around puberty in addition to the same muscular skeletal challenges that the boys have? What are the sports requirements of young female haemophiliacs who suffer profoundly heavy periods and are trying to participate in sports?

Globally, Haemophilia has the World Federation of Haemophilia and the European Haemophilia Consortium doing great work. Little Bleeders is different in being specifically about sport. Boys and girls will play football everywhere in the world whether they are healthy or not. In Senegal, haemophiliac boys are so desperate to play football with their friends that they do so without medication until they have a bleed and return to it as soon as they have recovered. They risk early death and guarantee later long-term debilitating injury, to join in the game they love. We are having conversations with the WFH and EHC about a partnership with their physical presence on the ground.

That side of my work protects me from the natural concerns of a retired athlete about becoming directionless without competitive sport in their life. I don't look ahead and worry about what I am going to do, and I don't look back and wish I had won more. As I said in Aguascalientes, everyone believed in me, I believed in me. And this was as far as I can go.

Is it weak of me to feel content and proud of my cycling career? Why would an athlete always think in terms of the losses, near misses, how good seven national titles would look compared to the six I have? I have been so blessed. Meeting Chanel, the birth of our daughter. My family and friends and teammates. All the injuries and near misses that could have been so much worse. The wins. It's a charmed life.

I know this doesn't fit the fist-pumping image of a professional sportsperson, but I feel happy with what I've done, and excited to bid the World Tour farewell and take up other sporting challenges where I can pursue my competitive instincts which remain, I assure you, as obsessively intense as ever.

My regrets are not the battles lost but the cumulative effect on Mum and Dad of all the battles, won or lost.

I once said to Dad when I was at Movistar, 'I've found a way to go faster.'

Dad said, 'Great. What is it, Alex?'

'I just hurt myself more or go to another level of pain.'

Dad looked crestfallen. Now that I am a father, I begin to understand why. There is no context in which a parent wants their child, whatever their age, to experience pain.

Mum has lived a life where everything stops if I am racing. Whether she is at the race or watching on TV, she combines a habit of shouting: 'Come on, Alex. Hurry up,' as if I'm late for dinner, with living in fear of me crashing. She watches all my races and hates every minute of it. Dad raced cars for a living but fears a bike pile-up way more than a car crash.

'When you retire, we do too,' he said to me, hinting at what they both go through.

Mum says I owe her a facelift.

A few days after telling Mum and Dad of my decision to retire from the World Tour, we had a conversation that began with Mum saying, 'If only we'd known at diagnosis how good it could be. How normal, how equal. If we could have taken away all the fear of those early times.'

I desperately want other parents of tiny haemophiliacs, in the dark days of diagnosis, to know what my parents didn't, that by being active and playing sport, your child can have the normal life that now seems like a dream.

But then the conversation took another direction. Dad suddenly looked upset. 'Alex,' he said. 'I need to ask you something.'

'Sure. What?'

'If you had your time again, and you now know what you missed out on with all your training and racing when your mates were having fun, would you not have done it?'

As he and Mum leaned closer, I realised that my answer to this was something big to them.

'I would do it all again,' I told them, not knowing if I was saying the right thing, but knowing I was saying the honest thing.

Dad breathed a big sigh of relief. He looked really happy. 'It's good to hear that.'

'What's this about?' I said.

'I've often felt sad you gave up your teenage years,' Mum said.

Dad said, 'I've worried I pushed you and you've missed out a normal life.'

'No,' I said. 'Absolutely not. I've loved it.'

And it's true. Even the bad times were a privilege.

'You're forgetting what you always said to me,' I said. '*If you wake us up, we'll take you.*'

That was the deal from the start. When I started swimming and felt my body growing strong, when I started to compete in the pool, the rule was that if I got myself up, and woke them, my parents would take me. It was clever of them. It meant me going would prove that I was wanting to do it, not that they were pushing me.

'You're forgetting that rule. You're forgetting that I wanted to do it.'

I was always self-motivated. Not everything about me comes from my disease, not by a long shot, but my determination to take part and to be strong was absolutely a response to a start in life that was about being in pain and being put on the sidelines. When I trained on the bike with Steve China at 6 a.m. on Saturday and Sunday mornings, when I was 16 and 17 and my mates were nursing a hangover, no one was getting me out of bed. I wanted to be doing it. I never skipped out on Steve and he never said, 'Well done' for turning up. Why should he, when he was turning up too? It was because he saw me doing all that, that Mum and Dad were happy to drive me up and down the country, and into Europe, to race. It was because I was committed that they were happy to find a way to buy me the bikes I needed.

Not only do I not regret it, I wanted it desperately. No one has forced me to do anything except to go to some races that I haven't necessarily thought were where I should go, but that's called having a job.

Elite athletes are selfish. Some are selfish and arseholes. Some are selfish and decent. But you get tired of everything in your life, as well as the lives of those close to you, being shaped by your own career, of rarely being free to drop everything for a friend, of constantly asking everyone else to make plans to fit around your training schedule. You know that most of them understand, that if you don't live and train like this, then pretty soon there will be nothing elite about you, but you reach a limit.

Leaving a stage of your career behind allows you to look at it from a different perspective and to appreciate it fully. I will miss the bunch because there is nothing like it. But I am not going to miss the near-death experience of the last half hour of most races. Cycling has changed a lot, and the talent that has been coming through had led me to a place where I have to put my hand up and say, 'I just can't be competitive often enough anymore.' It has been quite humbling.

Teams are shifting, understandably, to signing much younger riders. The World Tour has got harder with the younger style of racing. We saw it at my last Giro, which felt like a series of one-day races. I have never known a Giro like it. It was fun but brutally tough. We were dropping crazy power numbers just to remain in the game: 10 minutes at 450 Watts for me at 76kg was commonplace merely to hang in there. That's the evolution of the sport.

Chanel has listened to me talk about it, on and off, for a year. She has been the sympathetic ear who gave me the space to talk it through and to think aloud. If I had said to her: 'I think I can still compete, I still think I've still got this', she would have said, 'Great. What do we need to do to help you do it?' But what I have found myself saying is that I don't want to do it anymore. I've maxed myself out. There isn't anything better to come from me on the Tour. I think that's okay.

It's been heartbreaking watching some of my close friends on the World Tour go through painful and sometimes humiliating contract negotiations, and seeing others being forced into retirement. I found myself feeling happier and happier with making the decision to close this chapter and move to a new one. The flipside of the times we worry about the brevity of a sports career is now; being young, retired, with your life ahead of you and feeling excited about that, and hungry for new things. That's the transition of power from the known past to the unquantifiable future.

———

Ahead of the TT at my last Tour of Poland, my teammates and I were discussing who was going to win it. It was an 11km gradual uphill climb and most of the guys were saying it would be Ethan Hayter.

I said, 'Arensman.'

Thymen Arensman is a huge up-and-coming talent. He finished sixth when I was fifth in the TT at Tirreno–Adriatico 2022, one of my best-ever time trials and right at the end of my World Tour career. I had been aware of Thymen and impressed by him, but Tirreno was the first time I had beaten him and thought, *If I've beaten him, then I've definitely had a good ride.*

That thought process is part of the outgoing right-of-passage for a competitive sportsperson. Michael Hutchinson had the same thing with me. He heard about me, he beat me at races, he started noticing me, having battles with me and reached the point when beating me was not a given and meant something to him. Once I started beating him, I didn't stop. It's the natural way of time tapping on your shoulder.

I had never spoken to Thymen Arensman, but I sought him out in the peloton on Stage 5 in Poland, rode alongside him and said, 'Perfect TT for you tomorrow.'

He was coy. 'Oh, maybe, maybe, I hope so.'

Then we rode in silence for a while and I wondered if I'd done the wrong thing in seeking him out. I hadn't even said what I wanted to yet, which was that

I thought he was a fantastic talent and that I was really enjoying watching him progress.

'I can't believe you're talking to me,' Thymen said.

'What?'

'You're you. It's so nice you're talking to me.'

On my first Tour of Oman, with Livestrong in 2010, Filippo Pozzato helped me out with something that had come loose on my bike. He almost crashed trying to help me. Some of those older riders back then, like Fillipo and Tom Boonen, were so nice to me as a neo pro and I never forgot it.

'You don't realise how important you have been to my career,' Thymen said. 'Whenever you raced you've always put your numbers up on Strava, all the data, your power, everything. Most riders hide it all, just put up the route and their speed.'

I have never heard a convincing answer to why the data a cyclist produces should be hidden. I punched above my weight all my career when it comes to the results my amount of power should produce. No one gave me a reason not to share that data. But I was surprised, and chuffed, that this rider had got so much from it.

He said, 'When I was an U16 and junior I used to see your numbers and say to myself, that's what I'm aiming for to be pro. You were the only one who gave me that. You helped me so much.'

'Oh, well I'm surprised and so pleased,' I said . . .

. . . while wondering if Thymen Arensman was in fact the precise reason, finally, in human form, why I should never have shared my numbers. This talented, utterly polite and flattering young bastard had used them as a coaching tool and was now about to start beating me and then not stop beating me.

Another cue for retirement.

Thymen said some very generous things about my ride in Tirreno and what it had meant to him just to be in the mix with me. I wanted to tell him that Tirreno was the last time I would ever beat him, but I didn't want to put pressure on him. And I didn't want to sound in any way sad or regretful because, quite apart from the kind things he had said, listening to him had made me feel so positive about the future, his and mine.

'I hope you don't mind me saying, Thymen, but just keep doing what you're doing and being who you are.'

I think, and hope, he is going to be an outstanding racer and I am going to watch his career as a fan.

He won the time trial next day.

———

When you win, you understand that it's important to savour the moment, take it in, because life will move on quickly from it. I felt the same way about finishing on the World Tour throughout the second half of 2022. It was a chance, a fleeting one, to take stock of the Tour, the people on it, the life it gives you.

I've always loved having teammates. That includes everyone, soigneurs, mechanics, coaches, admin staff, as well as the riders. At Livestrong and Katusha, the people made the atmosphere fun and there was trust there. This was born out of pure youthful exuberance at Livestrong, and out of a them-versus-us bond among the riders at Katusha which developed as we watched things fall apart. Movistar were a team manager and a team with a beautiful spirit, which I probably did not integrate myself into as fully as I should have. When I think of that amazing day I broke the World Hour record with them in 2015, the way we celebrated, Eusebio's smile and bear hug for me as I came off the bike, I wonder if I appreciated them and him enough. I was young and ambitious and sometimes distracted.

It was an honour to start my career at Team Sky, to have two years there at my most formative stage, among the brilliant minds and talents that ran it and coached us. To begin my career in a team alongside Bradley Wiggins, Chris Froome and Geraint Thomas was an awesome experience.

But above all, the team of eight people who put together the Hour attempt in Mexico was the most special team I have ever been a part of. The day after it, as I sat in Aguascalientes airport at my lowest point, Mark Coyle sent the whole team a message that consisted solely of a quotation from Theodore Roosevelt:

> *It is not the critic who counts; not the man who points out how the strong man stumbles, or where the doer of deeds could have done them better. The*

credit belongs to the man who is actually in the arena, whose face is marred
by dust and sweat and blood; who strives valiantly; who errs, who comes short
again and again, because there is no effort without error and shortcoming;
but who does actually strive to do the deeds; who knows great enthusiasms, the
great devotions; who spends himself in a worthy cause; who at the best knows
in the end the triumph of high achievement, and who at the worst, if he fails,
at least fails while daring greatly, so that his place shall never be with those
cold and timid souls who neither know victory nor defeat.

Daylight is on the Andorran mountains and creeping into the valley. The flat is still silent. I love these quiet moments when I know my daughter and her mother are sound asleep. I use them to gain a little headspace and grow gradually more accustomed to no longer being Roosevelt's 'man in the arena'. I am so grateful to Chanel for helping me carve out time over the last year to work on this book. I'm grateful because it has allowed me the luxury of reflection at a crucial crossroads in my career, and the result is that I am now embarking on the next stage of my life not just with great optimism and a lot of ideas and ambition, but with profound thanks for all the years I was privileged to spend as a World Tour rider, for all the outstanding athletes I rode with and against, some geniuses among them. But most of all, I am grateful to have been able to think back to what my early life was like and to remind myself of the extraordinary thing my parents did for me in their darkest hour, when they led me to a life where anything is possible.

I was surrounded by legends, but they are my heroes.

ACKNOWLEDGEMENTS

Like many athletes, I am indebted to so many people for being a vital part of my journey. Some of them, like my coaches, family and mentors, know the part they have played. Others, by being a competitor or a friend, sometimes both, have helped me more than they realise. I have more people to thank than most due to the challenges my family and I faced in the early years

Firstly, I'd like to thank the incredible NHS, specifically Dan, Brian and the whole Haemophilia Team at the Royal London Hospital, for guiding us with a positive mindset, accepting road cycling instead of chess or a musical instrument, and expertly picking up the pieces when things went south.

I need to thank everyone working in those fields of medicine and science that pioneer ways for people like me with rare diseases to take our life expectancy from our teens to old age in a matter of a few short decades. I think about you and thank you every day.

To all my coaches, mentors, sponsors, teams, friends and supporters, you are the glue that held this journey together and developed it into something my family, doctors and I never believed possible back in 1990.

Thank you to Tom and Bloomsbury, for turning this unexpectedly wild ride into words I couldn't begin to articulate with such eloquence.

To my mum, dad and sister: Mum for her strength, love and steady hand with a needle; Dad for his positive outlook even when things looked bleak, and his ability to race so well that it filled a trophy cabinet that gave me inspiration and determination; and Lois, for being a best friend to me always, one who would even wear a helmet at the dinghy sailing club so I wasn't the only one. Thank you.

And finally thank you to Chanel, for going on that last-ditch attempt at a first date, for moving without hesitation to a country you'd never heard of simply because Rohan Dennis beat me by too much, for being so loving to Juliette and I, for being silly when silly is needed and serious when that is needed also, and for believing in me without question, even when you realised I wasn't the kind of professional cyclist that could deliver food to your front door. I love you. x

INDEX

INDEX